T0361797

Air Pollution and Health in Rapidly Developing Countries

Air Pollution and Health in Rapidly Developing Countries

EDITED BY
Gordon McGranahan
and Frank Murray

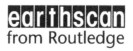

from Routledge

First published by Earthscan in the UK and USA in 2003

For a full list of publications please contact:

Earthscan
2 Park Square, Milton Park, Abingdon, Oxon OX14 4RN
Simultaneously published in the USA and Canada by Earthscan
711 Third Avenue, New York, NY 10017

Earthscan is an imprint of the Taylor & Francis Group, an informa business

Copyright © Stockholm Environment Institute, 2003

All rights reserved. No part of this book may be reprinted or reproduced or utilised in any form or by any electronic, mechanical, or other means, now known or hereafter invented, including photocopying and recording, or in any information storage or retrieval system, without permission in writing from the publishers.

Notices
Practitioners and researchers must always rely on their own experience and knowledge in evaluating and using any information, methods, compounds, or experiments described herein. In using such information or methods they should be mindful of their own safety and the safety of others, including parties for whom they have a professional responsibility.

Product or corporate names may be trademarks or registered trademarks, and are used only for identification and explanation without intent to infringe.

ISBN: 978-1-85383-985-6 (pbk)

Typesetting by MapSet Ltd, Gateshead, UK

Cover design by Declan Buckley

Library of Congress Cataloging-in-Publication Data

Air pollution and health in rapidly developing countries/[edited by] Gordon McGranahan, Frank Murray.
      p. cm.
   Includes bibliographical references and index.
   ISBN 1-85383-966-3 (hbk.) – ISBN 1-85383-985-X (pbk.).
   1. Air–Pollution–Health aspects–Developing countries. I. McGranahan, Gordon. II. Murray, Frank, 1950-

RA576.7.D44A37 2003
363.739'2'091724—dc21

2003003974

Contents

List of Figures

List of Tables

List of Contributors

Knut Aarhus is a political scientist conducting research and analysis on environmental policy and policy instruments at the ECON Centre for Economic Analysis in Oslo, Norway. He has conducted research and project assignments both nationally and internationally relating to the use of various policy instruments in the fields of energy and environment. He is presently working in the Performance Audit Department at the Office of the Auditor General in Norway, conducting performance audits of Norwegian development assistance.

Senior Adviser
Office of the Auditor General
PO Box 8130 Dep
0032 Oslo, Norway
Email: knut.aarhus@riksrevisjonen.no

Sameer Akbar has been working with the World Bank since August 1998. He has a postgraduate degree in mechanical engineering and undertook his doctoral research on particulate air pollution and health effects. At the World Bank he has been working on addressing environmental issues in projects and programmes, primarily in the energy and urban transport sectors. He also works on mainstreaming environmental issues at a strategic level in World Bank-aided policy reform and adjustment lending operations. He is currently responsible for managing the work programme on air pollution out of the India office of the World Bank. Before joining the World Bank he was conducting research at Imperial College, London.

Environmental Specialist
South Asia Environment and Social Development Unit
World Bank
70 Lodi Estate
New Delhi 110 003
India
Email: sakbar@worldbank.org

Fan Changzhong is an air pollution scientist and environmental impact assessment specialist conducting research and project assignments at the Guangzhou Research Institute of Environmental Protection at Guangzhou in China. He has conducted research oriented air quality management studies and projects in urban areas in Guangzhou and other places. He has published 20 articles in national and international journals. His research background is in air quality modelling and assessment methodologies, and the effective management of urban air pollution.

Director
Environmental Impact Assessment (EIA) Division
Guangzhou Research Institute of Environmental Protection
24 Nanyi Road, Tianhe Guangzhou, PR China (Post Code: 510620)
Email: fanchangzhong@163.com

Anthony Johnson Hedley is a graduate in medicine of the universities of Aberdeen and Edinburgh. In his early career he specialized in internal medicine and endocrinology before moving to the field of public health and preventive medicine. He was professor of public health at the University of Glasgow from 1983 to 1988, and in 1988 became head of the Department of Community Medicine at the University of Hong Kong and honorary consultant to the Department of Health and the Hospital Authority. His main areas of interest and research include tobacco control, the health effects of air pollution, the evaluation of healthcare delivery and postgraduate medical education.

Department of Community Medicine
The University of Hong Kong
5/F, Academic and Administration Block
Faculty of Medicine Building
21 Sassoon Road, Hong Kong
Email: commed@hkucc.hku.hk

Mauricio Hernandez-Avila is an epidemiologist with extensive experience in research and human resource development in Latin America. With degrees in medicine, pathology, statistics, applied mathematics and epidemiology, One of the foremost pioneers of epidemiology in Mexico, he began work as the Director of Epidemiological Surveillance, Chronic Diseases and Accidents in the General Directorate of Epidemiology, filling this post from 1988 to 1991. In 1991 he became the director of the Center for Population Health Research at the National Institute of Public Health. He has consolidated an inter-institutional group that develops research on environmental pollution in relation to lead intoxication and air pollution health effects.

Director General
Center for Population Research
National Institute of Public Health
Av Universidad #655
Cuernavaca, Morelos, MEXICO
Email: mhernan@correo.insp.mx

Huib Jansen is an environmental economist. Until his retirement in 2000, he was associated with the Institute for Environmental Studies at the Vrije Universiteit Amsterdam. He has performed many studies for many national and international commissioners, such as UNEP, the European Commission and the World Bank. He was also the executive managing editor of the journal *Environmental and Resource Economics.*

Former Senior Researcher at the Institute for Environmental Studies,
Vrije Universiteit Amsterdam
Le Bourg
24250 Daglan, France
Email: Catherine.jansen@wanadoo.fr

Tai-Hing Lam is Chair Professor and Head of Department of Community Medicine at the University of Hong Kong. Professor Lam's research interests include family planning and youth sexuality, the epidemiology of cancer, cardiovascular and respiratory diseases and their risk factors, health services research with a major focus on tobacco-related diseases, tobacco control measures and smoking cessation. Professor Lam has produced over 300 publications and presentations, including papers in major journals such as the *Lancet*, the *British Medical Journal* and the *Journal of the American Medical Association.* Professor Lam was awarded a commemorative certificate and medal by the World Health Organization in May 1998 for achievements worthy of international recognition in promoting the concept of tobacco-free societies.

Department of Community Medicine
The University of Hong Kong
5/F, Academic and Administration Block
Faculty of Medicine Building
21 Sassoon Road, Hong Kong
Email: commed@hkucc.hku.hk

Steinar Larssen is an air pollution scientist and air quality management specialist conducting research and project assignments at the Norwegian Institute for Air Research at Kjeller in Norway. He is a consultant and expert adviser to several international agencies, including the European Environment Agency, the World Bank and the Norwegian Agency for Development Cooperation. He has conducted research-oriented air quality management studies and projects in urban areas in South and East Asian countries as well as in other regions. His research background is in air quality monitoring and assessment methodologies and the effective management of urban air pollution.

Associate Research Director
Norwegian Institute for Air Research
2010 Kjeller, Norway
Email: Steinar.Larssen@nilu.no

Morton Lippmann is an environmental health scientist conducting research into human exposure to airborne toxicants and their health effects at New York University's Nelson Institute of Environmental Medicine. His academic duties include graduate and postgraduate teaching and research guidance. He has chaired the US Environmental Protection Agency's Science Advisory Board, Clean Air Scientific Advisory Committee, Human Exposure Committee and Dioxin and Related Compound Risk Assessment Review Committee, as well as the NIOSH Board of Scientific Counselors and the External Scientific Advisory Committees for the Southern California Children's Health Study of air pollution at the University of Southern California, and the National Environmental Respiratory Center study of the toxicology of source-related air pollutant mixtures in Albuquerque.

Professor of Environmental Medicine
New York University School of Medicine
Nelson Institute of Environmental Medicine
57 Old Forge Road
Tuxedo, NY 10987, USA
Email: lippmann@env.med.nyu.edu

Stefan Ma has Bachelors and Masters degrees in statistics. He worked for six and a half years for the Department of Community Medicine at the University of Hong Kong, and for two years in a managed care company in Hong Kong, before moving to the Ministry of Health in Singapore in 2001. He provided the statistical input for studying air pollution effects on health in the department. His current main areas of interest are health inequality, disease projection and estimations of disease burden.

Biostatistics and Research Branch
Epidemiology and Disease Control Division
Ministry of Health, College of Medicine Building
16 College Road, Singapore 169854
Email: stefan_ma@moh.gov.sg

Sarah Morag McGhee is a health services researcher with a particular interest in applications of economic methods. She carries out research and teaching at the University of Hong Kong and is currently a member of the Hong Kong SAR Government Expert Sub-committee on Grant Applications and Awards and the Cervical Screening Task Force. She has also carried out research work for the government's Environmental Protection Department, the Health and Welfare Bureau and the Hospital Authority. She has an honorary membership of the UK Faculty of Public Health Medicine. She has recently carried out work in costing air pollution and tobacco-related disease.

Associate Professor
Department of Community Medicine, University of Hong Kong
5/F Academic and Administrative Block, Faculty of Medicine Building
21 Sassoon Road, Hong Kong
Email: smmcghee@hkucc.hku.hk

Gordon McGranahan is currently Director of the Human Settlements Programme at the International Institute for Environment and Development. Trained as an economist, he spent the 1990s at the Stockholm Environment Institute, where he directed the Urban Environment Programme and coordinated an international study of local environment and health problems in low and middle income cities. He has also worked for the World Bank and Brookhaven National Laboratory. He has published widely on urban environmental issues and was the first author of a recent book entitled *The Citizens at Risk: From Urban Sanitation to Sustainable Cities* (Earthscan, 2001).

Director
Human Settlements Programme
International Institute for Environment and Development
3 Endsleigh Street
London WC1H 0DD
United Kingdom
Email: gordon.mcgranahan@iied.org

Angela Mathee heads the Environment and Health Research Office at the South African Medical Research Council. She is also a member of the Executive Committee of the Public Health Association of South Africa, and has served as adviser to the World Health Organization in respect of air pollution in African cities and environment and health in sustainable development. Previously she held the position of Executive Officer for Urban Environmental Management at the Greater Johannesburg (Eastern) Metropolitan Local Council. Her main research interests relate to ambient and indoor air pollution, housing and childhood lead exposure in developing countries.

Senior Specialist Scientist
Environmental Health
South African Medical Research Council
PO Box 87373, Houghton, 2041, South Africa
Email: amathee@mrc.ac.za

Frank Murray is an environmental scientist conducting research and teaching in the School of Environmental Science, Murdoch University, Perth, Australia. He is also a member of a number of government policy committees and boards, including the Environmental Protection Authority, a five-member statutory authority responsible for environmental policy development and environmental impact assessment. He is a consultant and expert adviser to several international agencies. His research background is in air quality monitoring and management and the effects of air pollution.

Associate Professor in Environmental Systems
School of Environmental Science
Division of Science and Engineering
Murdoch University, Murdoch WA 6150, Australia
Email: F. Murray@murdoch.edu.au

Xander A Olsthoorn is a senior researcher associated with the Institute for Environmental Studies at the Vrije Universiteit Amsterdam. He trained as a chemical engineer. Most of his work is performed in a multidisciplinary context, in particular in cooperation with economists and social scientists. His main research areas are the assessment of the economic impacts of air pollution and the analysis of the climate change-related socio-economic impacts of extreme weather events.

Senior Researcher
Institute for Environmental Studies
Vrije Universiteit Amsterdam
De Boelelaan 1087
1081 HV Amsterdam
Email: Xander.Olsthoorn@ivm.vu.nl

Bart D Ostro is currently the Chief of the Air Pollution Epidemiology Unit, Office of Environmental Health Hazard Assessment, California Environmental Protection Agency. His primary responsibilities are to formulate the agency's recommendations for state ambient air quality standards and to investigate the potential health effects of criteria air pollutants (such as particulate matter, ozone and lead). His previous research has contributed to the determination of federal and state air pollution standards for ozone and particulate matter and he was co-author of the EPA analysis that led to the federal ban on lead in gasoline. Dr Ostro has served as a consultant with several institutions (including the US Environmental Protection Agency, the Departments of State and Energy, the East–West Center, the World Health Organization, the World Bank and the Asian Development Bank) and with foreign governments including those of Mexico, Indonesia, Thailand and Chile. He currently serves on a National Academy of Science Committee on Quantifying the Benefits of Air Pollution Control.

Chief
Air Pollution Epidemiology Unit
California Office of Environmental Health Hazard Assessment (OEHHA)
1515 Clay St, 16th Floor
Oakland, CA 94612
Email: Bostro@oehha.ca.gov

Isabelle Romieu is a medical epidemiologist whose primary interest lies in environmental health in Latin American countries, particularly the adverse effects of air pollution and other environmental agents on children's respiratory health. She has worked in the Latin American region for 12 years with the Pan American Health Organization on human resource development and institutional strengthening in environmental health, as well as carrying out research projects concerning children's health, such as the impact of vehicular traffic and the corresponding risk of asthma in children. She has spearheaded numerous regional projects concerning children's health in the Americas, such as a Pan-American Lead Workshop in Peru (2001) and a Pediatric

Environmental Health Specialty Unit in Mexico. She is presently Professor of Environmental Epidemiology at the National Institute of Public Health in Mexico, and serves as consultant and expert adviser to several international and governmental organizations.

Associate Professor in Environmental Epidemiology
National Institute of Public Health (INSP)
Av Universidad #655
Col Sta Ma Ahuacatitlan
62508 Cuernavaca Morelos
Mexico
Email: iromieu@correo.insp.mx

Sumeet Saksena conducts research on human exposure to air pollution in developing countries. He has experience in field and policy research in Asian countries. He is currently studying the role of uncertainty in exposure estimates in policy formulation. He has worked on projects and consultancy assignments funded by various UN agencies. He is a member of many international societies, committees and boards.

Fellow
East–West Center
1601 East–West Center
Honolulu, HI 96848
USA
Email: saksenas@eastwestcenter.org

Dietrich Schwela is responsible for the normative work of the World Health Organization (WHO) (Headquarters) in air quality and health (WHO guidelines for air quality, WHO guidelines for community noise, WHO-UNEP-WMO health guidelines for vegetation fire events, WHO guidelines for biological agents in the indoor environment); for networking within the Air Management Information System; for the evidence-based estimation of the global, regional and local burden of disease due to air pollution; for intervention support (prevention, mitigation and reduction of the burden of disease due to long term and short term exposure to air pollution); and for capacity building (regional and national training workshops in air quality and health). He is a member of several scientific bodies.

Air Pollution Scientist
Occupational and Environmental Health
Department of Protection of the Human Environment
World Health Organization
20 Avenue Appia, CH-1211
Geneva 20, Switzerland
Email: schwelad@who.int

Jitendra J Shah is an environmental engineer at the World Bank. He has over 25 years of research and project management experience in the US and internationally. At the World Bank, his work ranges from conceptualization to the implementation of regional air quality programmes to deal with issues such as acid rain in Asia and urban air quality management. He manages some of the environmental investment projects that deal with ozone hole protection and global climate change. He also assists with and reviews the environmental impact assessment of Bank-financed projects. His research background is in air quality modelling, policy analysis and transferring international experiences to developing countries.

Senior Environmental Engineer
World Bank
1818 H St NW
Washington, DC 20433, USA
Email: Jshah@worldbank.org

Kirk R Smith conducts research and teaching on the relationships between environment, development and health in developing countries. He has worked extensively on air pollution problems in Asia and Latin America, both indoor and outdoor, urban and rural, and health-damaging and climate-warming. He sits on a number of national and international advisory boards and the editorial boards of several international scientific journals. He is most well known for his pioneering work, begun in 1980, to elucidate the health impacts of indoor air pollution in developing countries from the use of solid household fuels.

Professor and Chair, Environmental Health Sciences
School of Public Health
University of California
Berkeley, California 94720-7360, USA
Email: krksmith@uclink.berkeley.edu

Yasmin von Schirnding is the focal point for Agenda 21 at the World Health Organization, and WHO's representative on the Inter-Agency Committee on Sustainable Development. She is based in the Director-General's Office where she is responsible for cross-sectoral policies and interventions relating to health and sustainable development. She was previously responsible for the Office of Global and Integrated Environmental Health at WHO. Prior to coming to WHO she was Director of Environmental Health for Johannesburg. She is a past and current member of a wide range of professional bodies including the International Society for Environmental Epidemiology, in which she served as an elected councillor on the board. She has a particular interest in bridging the gaps between health, environment and development policies, strategies and practices, and has published widely in the field of health, environment and sustainable development.

Focal Point: Agenda 21
Strategy Unit
Office of the Director General
World Health Organization
20 Avenue Appia
CH-1211 Geneva 27
Switzerland
Email: vonschirndingy@who.ch

Michael P Walsh is a mechanical engineer who has spent his entire career working on motor vehicle pollution control issues at the local, national and international levels. During the 1980s he was an adviser to the US Senate Environment and Public Works Committee during development of the 1990 Clean Air Act amendments. He currently co-chairs the US Environmental Protection Agency's Mobile Source Advisory Subcommittee and is actively involved in projects in Brazil, Hong Kong, Moscow and China. He is also a member of the National Research Council Committee on the Future of Personal Transport Vehicles in China. He is the principal technical consultant to the Asian Development Bank regarding a regional technical assistance project, Reducing Motor Vehicle Emissions in Asia, and served as a peer review expert to the EU Commission during its recent deliberations regarding near zero sulphur fuels. He was selected as the first recipient of the US Environmental Protection Agency Lifetime Individual Achievement Award for 'outstanding achievement, demonstrated leadership and a lasting commitment to promoting clean air'.

3105 North Dinwiddie Street
Arlington, VA 22207
USA
Email: mpwalsh@igc.org

Chit-Ming Wong is a statistician undertaking research and teaching in the Department of Community Medicine, University of Hong Kong. He is a member of the government Sub-Working Group on the Review of Hong Kong's Air Quality Objectives. He is a statistical referee of the government Expert Sub-Committee on Grant Applications and Awards, the *Hong Kong Medical Journal* and the *International Journal of Epidemiology*. His research background is in the health effects of air pollution, statistical modelling and health needs measures.

Assistant Professor in Biostatistics
Department of Community Medicine
University of Hong Kong
5/F, Academic and Administration Block
Faculty of Medicine Building
21 Sassoon Road
Hong Kong
Email: hrmrwcm@hkucc.hku.hk

Preface

The global environment is changing rapidly, partly in response to economic globalization. These global changes are clearly evident at the local level, even in the quality of air that people breath. In some high income countries air quality has been improving, due to a combination of de-industrialization, improved technologies and environmental regulation. However, advances in the science of epidemiology suggest that even air that would until recently have been considered 'clean' may contain pollutants that are hazardous to people's health. Moreover, in many low and middle income countries, economic growth is still associated with declining air quality.

The enormous toll on human health and the environment imposed by early industrialization in Europe and North America has been well documented. We now know far more about how uncontrolled industrialization and motorization results in increased emissions and discharges that eventually expose people to hazardous pollutants. In some countries it seems that the failings of early industrialization are nevertheless being repeated. In others, the early introduction and enforcement of appropriate policies are making a positive difference. It is important to learn not only from past mistakes, but also from more recent successes.

There are many factors involved in the development and effective implementation of policies to achieve sustainable development, and many difficult decisions have to be taken in the allocation of scarce resources. This book seeks to examine a component of the wider problem. It focuses on the issue of air pollution and health in developing nations. It examines aspects of what we have learned about air pollution and health, and the consequences for health of improvements in air quality. As most of this information has been gained in relatively wealthy cities, this book addresses important questions relating to the applicability of what we have learned in relatively wealthy cities to the situation faced by low and middle income cities.

Considerable knowledge about the consequences of air pollution on health has been gained, especially in recent years, but much of this knowledge has not been made available in a form accessible beyond some scientific disciplines. This book aims to make some of this knowledge accessible to a wider audience.

Many attempts have been made to control air pollution and improve air quality around the world. Rapid improvements in technology and the introduction of new policy ideas have led to new tools that may be applied to improve air quality. Some of these tools are also described.

Even in low and middle income cities there is enormous diversity, not only in air pollution problems but in opportunities for improvement. This means that the lessons of science and policy need to be adapted to a wide range of settings, as illustrated in examples provided throughout the book.

While the human population of the planet continues to increase, and the differences in wealth and consumption continue to grow, the physical resources of the planet are finite. Globalization has made it increasingly obvious that we live in a global village, and it is in the interests of all villagers, rich or poor, to ensure that the planet that sustains us is healthy. The analyses reported on in this book provide important elements of the knowledge base for the actions needed to make the planet healthier.

Roger Kasperson
Executive Director
Stockholm Environment Institute
July 2002

List of Acronyms and Abbreviations

$\mu g/m^3$	micrograms per cubic metre
μm	micrometre (a millionth of a metre)
A	attributable proportion
ABNT	Associação Brasileira de Normas Técnicas (Brazil)
ACS	American Cancer Society
AEA	Atomic Energy Agency
ALRI	acute lower respiratory infection
AMIS	Air Management Information System (World Health Organization)
ANFAVEA	Associação Nacional dos Fabricantes de Veículos Automotores
APHEA	Air Pollution on Health: a European Approach
AQIS	Air Quality Information System
AQMS	air quality management strategy
AQO	air quality objective
ARI	acute respiratory infection
Beijing EPB	Beijing Municipal Environment Protection Bureau
BMU	German Federal Environment Agency
BS	black smoke
BTT	birth-to-ten (research project)
CAIP	clean air implementation plan
CBA	cost–benefit analysis
CEC	Commission of the European Communities
CETESB	Companhia de Tecnologia de Saneamento Ambiental (Brazil)
CI	confidence interval
CNG	compressed natural gas
CNS	central nervous system
CO	carbon monoxide
CO_2	carbon dioxide
CONAMA	Conselho Nacional do Meio Ambiente (Brazil)
CONMETRO	Conselho Nacional de Metrologia, Normalização e Qualidade Industrial (Brazil)
CONTRAN	Conselho Nacional de Trânsito (Brazil)
COPD	chronic obstructive pulmonary disease
CP	coarse particles
CSIR	Council for Scientific and Industrial Research
DSS IPC	Decision Support System for Industrial Pollution Control
EIA	environmental impact assessment
EPA	Environmental Protection Agency (US)

ERV	emergency room visit
EU	European Union
EU CAFE	European Union Clean Air for Europe Programme
FEV	forced expiratory volume
FEV_1	forced expiratory volume in the first second of a vital capacity manoeuvre
FGD	flue gas desulphurization
FS	fuel switch
FVC	forced vital capacity
GAM	generalized additive model
GDP	gross domestic product
GEMS/AIR	Global Environmental Monitoring System
GHG	greenhouse gas
GIS	Geographical Information Systems
GJMC	Greater Johannesburg Metropolitan Council
GOI	Government of India
GRIEP	Guangzhou Research Institute for Environmental Protection
GWC	global warming commitment
H_2SO_4	sulphuric acid
HC	hydrocarbons
HDP	health-damaging pollutants
HDV	heavy duty vehicle
HEI	Health Effects Institute
HIV	human immunodeficiency virus
HKSAR	Hong Kong Special Administrative Region
HNO_3	nitric acid
HSU	Hartridge Smoke Unit
IARC	International Agency for Research on Cancer
IBAMA	Instituto Nacional do Meio Ambiente e dos Recursos Naturais Renováveis (Brazil)
INMETRO	Instituto Nacional de Metrologia, Normalização e Qualidade Industrial (Brazil)
IRIS	Integrated Risk Information System (US EPA)
IVL	Swedish Environmental Research Institute
LDV	light duty vehicle
LNB	low NO_x burner
LPG	liquefied petroleum gas
LS	low sulphur
MARC	Monitoring and Assessment Research Centre
MATES	Multiple Air Toxics Exposure Study
MMVF	manmade vitreous fibre
MRT	mass rapid transit (Singapore)
MSAT	mobile source air toxics
MW	megawatt
NAAQS	National Ambient Air Quality Standards (US)
NAFTA	North American Free Trade Area
NH_3	ammonia

NILU	Norsk Institut for Luftforskning (Norwegian Institute for Air Research)
NO	nitric oxide
NO_2	nitrogen dioxide
NO_3	nitrate
NORAD	Norwegian Department of Foreign Aid and Development
NO_x	nitrogen oxides
NYU	New York University
O_3	ozone
OBD	Onboard Diagnostics
OECD	Organisation for Economic Co-operation and Development
OFA	over-fire air
PAH	polycyclic aromatic hydrocarbons
PAHO	Pan American Health Organization
PAN	peroxyacetyl nitrate
PCB	polychlorinated biphenyl
PEFR	peak expiratory flow rate
PM	particulate matter
PM_{10}	fine particles with aerodynamic diameters less than 10µm
$PM_{2.5}$	fine particles with aerodynamic diameters less than 2.5µm
POM	polycyclic organic matter
ppb	parts per billion
ppm	parts per million
PROCONVE	Programa de Controle da Poluição por Veículos Automotores (Brazil)
RAD	restricted activity days
RAPIDC	Regional Air Pollution in Developing Countries (programme)
REA	rapid epidemiological assessment
RfC	reference concentration
RfD	reference dose
RHA	respiratory hospital admission
RR	relative risk
RSD	respiratory symptom day
RSP	respirable suspended particulates
SCR	selective catalytic reduction
SEARO	South-East Asia Regional Office
SEI	Stockholm Environment Institute
SEMA	Secretaria Especial do Meio Ambiente (Brazil)
SI	sorbent injection
SIAM	Society of Indian Automobile Manufacturers
Sida	Swedish International Development Cooperation Agency
SO_2	sulphur dioxide
SO_4	sulphate
SO_x	sulphur oxide
SPM	suspended particulate matter
SPMR	Sao Paulo Metropolitan Region
TB	tuberculosis

TOG	total organic gases
TSP	total suspended particulate matter
TWC	three-way catalytic converters
UAQM	urban air quality management
UN/ECE	United Nations Economic Commission for Europe
UNEP	United Nations Environment Programme
URBAIR	Urban Air Quality Management Strategy (World Bank project)
UV	ultraviolet
VOC	volatile organic compound
VSL	value of a statistical life
WB	World Bank
WHO	World Health Organization
WHO-EURO	World Health Organization Regional Office for Europe
WMO	World Meteorological Organization
WRAC	wide ranging aerosol classifier
WTP	willingness to pay

Acknowledgements

The work contained in this book is multidisciplinary. It attempts to synthesize information from a range of disciplines, many of which have reductionist structures and high barriers separating them. The results of work in these disciplines are normally communicated to those within the discipline, and relatively infrequently to a broader community.

In preparing this book the authors of chapters, and we as editors, have tried to balance the need to maintain the integrity of the language and understandings within specific disciplines with the use of more general terms (and sometimes generalizations) that are required to synthesize knowledge from different disciplines and make this knowledge available to a wider audience. This synthesis is a balancing act, and if we as editors have made errors and dropped a few plates along the way, we apologize and ask for understanding from all those disciplines we may have transgressed. For such omissions, misunderstandings and transgressions, please do not punish the authors of chapters. They were acting under orders.

The work contained in this book was coordinated by the Stockholm Environment Institute (SEI) and funded by the Swedish International Development Cooperation Agency (Sida) over a number of years. The work is part of the programme on Regional Air Pollution In Developing Countries (RAPIDC). A large number of people have contributed to the work. These include Vikrom Mathur, Steve Cinderby, Kevin Hicks and Katarina Axelsson of SEI, and especially Johan Kuylenstierna, who provided enormous encouragement and advice during the development, planning and execution of this work.

Much of the information presented in this publication was discussed at a workshop held in Hyderabad and attended by participants from India, Pakistan, Nepal, Sri Lanka and Bangladesh, who provided very useful discussion and commentary. We would like to thank all of those who attended the workshop and in particular the workshop organizers: M G Gopal of the Environmental Protection Training Research Institute, Hyderabad, India; Raghunathan Rajamani, Mylvakanam Iyngararasan and Surendra Shrestha of the United Nations Environment Programme Environmental Assessment Programme for Asia and the Pacific; and Pradyumna Kumar Kotta and Ananda Raj Joshi of the South Asia Cooperative Environmental Programme.

We would like to thank the authors, who gave up so much time to produce the chapters within this book, their colleagues and their families.

We would especially like to acknowledge the cheerful hard work and long hours of Isobel Devane and Lisetta Tripodi, who read and corrected very many errors we provided, and Erik Willis for the fine job he did with the figures.

Frank Murray and *Gordon McGranahan*
Perth, Australia, and London
June 2002

Introduction

Air Pollution and Health in Developing Countries – The Context

Frank Murray and Gordon McGranahan

OBJECTIVES

The aim of this book is to synthesize policy-relevant knowledge on air pollution and health, and thereby provide a firmer basis for improving public health in low and middle income countries. The information presented is of particular relevance to middle income countries, where urban concentrations of health-damaging pollutants are often among the highest in the world, and preventive and protective measures are still at an early stage. It is also relevant to low income countries, where air pollution problems tend to be more localized, but can be very severe when they do arise.

Recent decades have seen considerable progress in the epidemiology of air pollution, significant changes in international air pollution guidelines and the emergence of more systematic approaches to air pollution control. Many of these advances have originated in affluent countries and regions, but there have also been important developments in many other parts of the world. This publication seeks to make these advances accessible to a wider audience including, especially, those concerned with developing or supporting locally driven processes of air pollution management.

The chapters that follow cover a range of topics relevant to local air pollution management. Studies from Europe and North America, where the research is comparatively advanced, are reviewed to provide insights into the relationships between some of the most critical air pollutants and health. Studies from a wide range of less heavily researched Asian, African and Latin American countries are also reviewed, and the findings are contrasted with those from Europe and North America. Various tools and systems for air pollution management are described, with an emphasis on approaches that can be used when data are scarce. Two issues of particular relevance to low and middle income countries – indoor air pollution and vehicular pollution – are examined in more detail. In addition, a small selection of case studies – one from Asia, one from Africa and one from Latin America – are summarized.

In most chapters the emphasis is on the scientific and technical aspects of air pollution and health policy. Comparatively little attention is given to the politics, economics or non-health social implications of air pollution. This should not be taken to imply that air pollution management is or should become a technical exercise that is divorced from local politics. Indeed, as many chapters make clear, air pollution management is ultimately a political process, with economic as well as health implications and a wide range of stakeholders. A better understanding of the relations between air pollution and health, air pollution guidelines, and more systematic approaches to air pollution control can all contribute to, but never replace, political debate and good governance.

In the following sections of this chapter background information is provided on the historical context of air pollution, some of the more widely relevant types and sources of air pollution and the policy issues that motivated this publication. The Introduction ends with a summary of the contents of the later chapters.

Air pollution in its Historical Context

Air pollution may be defined as the presence of substances in air at concentrations, durations and frequencies that adversely affect human health, human welfare or the environment. Air pollution is not a recent phenomenon. The remains of early humans demonstrate that they suffered the detrimental effects of smoke in their dwellings (Brimblecombe, 1987). Blackening of lung tissues through long exposure to particulate air pollution in smoky dwellings appears to be common in mummified lung tissue from ancient humans. Unhealthy air was a suspected cause of disease long before the relationship could be scientifically confirmed. Indeed, the miasma theory of disease, still widely held well into the 19th century, blamed a wide range of health problems on bodily disturbances resulting from 'bad' air.

It was with industrialization that local impacts of air pollution on human health and the environment began to be documented systematically. However, industrialization also fostered the idea that air pollution was a necessary product of economic development. Partly as a result, mounting evidence of serious air pollution problems did not initially provide the basis for decisive action.

Statistics were collected on deaths resulting from air pollution in the 18th and 19th centuries and in the early part of the 20th century in London; in the Meuse Valley, Belgium; Donora, US; New York City, US; Osaka, Japan; and elsewhere (see Table I.1). A number of cities introduced smoke control ordinances around the turn of the 20th century, and by 1912, 23 of the largest 25 cities in the US had ordinances principally aimed at visible smoke from commercial establishments (Tarr, 1996). High air pollution levels persisted in many of the major cities of Europe and North America, and during five days in December 1952 it is estimated that there were about 4000 excess deaths

Table I.1 *Some major air pollution episodes and associated deaths*

Date	Place	Excess deaths
December 1873	London, UK	270–700
February 1880	London, UK	1000
December 1892	London, UK	1000
December 1930	Meuse Valley, Belgium	63
October 1948	Donora, US	20
December 1952	London, UK	4000
November 1953	New York City, US	250
January 1956	London, UK	480
December 1957	London, UK	300–800
November–December 1962	New York City, US	46
December 1962	London, UK	340–700
December 1962	Osaka, Japan	60
January–February 1963	New York City, US	200–405
November 1966	New York City, US	168

Source: after Elsom, 1992

in London from a stagnant atmosphere of fog, smoke and sulphur dioxide (Brimblecombe, 1987). Epidemiological studies of air pollution and health only really began in earnest after this London episode.

Over the course of the 20th century, attitudes and policies towards air pollution were slowly shifting, however, and in many affluent cities air pollution levels declined. As evidence on the health risks accumulated, public concern about the dangers of air pollution grew. As more efficient and clean fuels became available, industrial smoke ceased to be associated with progress and modern technology. As incomes increased and the costs of cleaner technologies and fuels fell, air pollution control became less economically onerous.

In the early stages air pollution measures emphasized the more visible and immediate pollution, such as the particulate and sulphur dioxide concentrations in cities. These measures included the location of heavy industry outside population centres, and the requirement for major emission sources to discharge from tall chimneys to disperse the emissions and thus reduce ground level concentrations. However, some of these measures contributed to regional air pollution, as emissions from urban and industrial areas can travel long distances, crossing national boundaries and affecting health and environments in rural areas and in other countries.

In response, more effective international action was eventually implemented. International guidelines on ambient air quality have been produced by organizations such as the World Health Organization (WHO) (WHO, 2000a, 2000b), and international policies are being coordinated under conventions such as the Convention on Long-range Transboundary Air Pollution (UN ECE, 1995).

In the last two or three decades attention in high income countries has been broadened to include reducing emissions of carbon monoxide, hydrocarbons, nitrogen oxides, toxic compounds, lead and other heavy metals, although the emphasis and success of management activities have varied in different places at different times. Increasing attention is also being given to reducing exposure to indoor air pollutants and, at the other end of the scale, reducing emissions of greenhouse gases (GHGs).

Partly as a result of this history, most of the published studies on the effects on human health of air pollution relate to the effects of outdoor air pollution on residents of North America and Europe of Caucasian descent, usually of good nutritional status, living in uncrowded conditions, without physical stress or untreated chronic diseases. There are relatively few studies on populations of other ethnic backgrounds, nutritional status, living conditions, stress or history of chronic diseases, or of indoor air pollution. These factors may alter the dose–response relations derived for exposure to outdoor air pollutants (WHO, 2000b).

The current relationship between economic affluence and health-threatening ambient air pollution involves a number of opposing tendencies. For example, industrialization and motorization tend to increase the level of potentially polluting activities. Greater affluence, on the other hand, provides an increasing capacity to monitor and control pollution (as well as leading, after a certain point, to a structural shift in a national economy away from the more polluting activities, the products of which can be imported from middle income countries). The first tendency appears to dominate at lower income levels, while the second dominates at the upper end. Thus studies have found that urban sulphur dioxide concentrations tend to increase with economic development, and then to decline as air pollution controls become more stringent (Grossman and Krueger, 1995; Shafik, 1995). There are indications that some other health-threatening pollutants, such as coarse particulates and lead, follow similar patterns. Overall, the worst ambient air pollution problems are often located in industrialized cities in middle income countries.

Indoor air pollution tends to decline with economic affluence, since smoky cooking and heating fuels are the major sources of indoor pollution, and are used mostly by low income households. Indoor air pollution is a particular problem in low income rural areas, where fuelwood and biofuels are plentiful and people cannot easily afford cleaner fuels. When polluting household fuels are used in urban areas, they can also contribute significantly to ambient air pollution, particularly in and around low income neighbourhoods (Krzyzanowski and Schwela, 1999).

Emissions of GHGs are often associated with emissions of other air pollutants and tend to increase with economic growth, since economic activity is still heavily dependent on the fossil fuels that account for most carbon emissions. The health effects of climate change are complex, delayed and far beyond the scope of this book. The global agreements necessary to address GHG emissions are still being developed. On the other hand, the international politics and economics of climate change are already beginning to influence local policy debates surrounding air pollution and health. From the perspective of low and middle income countries, for example, it is critical that measures to reduce carbon emissions (undertaken, for example, through the Clean Development Mechanism) also result in reduced exposure to hazardous pollutants.

At every level of economic development, ambient air pollution poses a serious challenge that cannot be left to private initiatives, even in established market economies. There are a number of reasons why air pollution problems tend to be ignored in private negotiation and decision-making. The damage caused by air pollution is often difficult to perceive, even when the effects are substantial, and people rarely know the levels or sources of the pollution they are being exposed to. Even if they did know, there are no markets through which to negotiate reductions in air pollution (in economic terms, air pollution is an externality). And even if there were markets for clean air, they would not operate efficiently, since many of the benefits of better air quality are public and cannot be bought and sold on an individual basis (again, in economic terms, clean air is a public good). It is no coincidence that economists often use air pollution examples to help describe the different forms of 'market failure'. Without effective policies, supported by good science, air pollution will tend to be excessive at every level.

Especially in low and middle income countries, governments also have difficulty coming to terms with air pollution and health problems. The overall extent of air pollution problems is often poorly understood. The information and policy tools needed to take effective action are often lacking. There are well founded concerns that inappropriate air pollution controls can inhibit economic growth, alongside unfounded concerns that even well designed air pollution policies are anti-growth. The few who might be seriously hurt by air pollution controls are often more vocal and influential than the many who could benefit. In the absence of public pressure, governments too are inclined to ignore air pollution problems.

Both public and governmental concerns about air pollution are increasing, however, and significant actions to improve air quality are increasingly evident in middle income countries. It would be inappropriate for low and middle income countries to adopt the air pollution policies of high income countries. It would be equally inappropriate for them to replicate the very slow process of air pollution policy development that occurred historically in high income countries. If the emerging debates about air pollution and health are to lead to effective policies, it is critical that they be locally driven. However, it is also critical that they be internationally informed. There is a great deal to learn, not only from the science of air pollution but also from the approaches to air pollution management that have been adopted in different parts of the world.

TYPES AND SOURCES OF AIR POLLUTION

There is a wide range of pollutants present in indoor and outdoor air. They include many types of particulates, sulphur oxides, carbon monoxide, ozone and other photochemical oxidants, nitrogen oxides, toxic compounds, lead and other heavy metals, and a variety of volatile organic compounds (VOCs). Due to the many differences in the sources, distribution and effects of these compounds, to avoid overgeneralization it is preferable to treat them separately. However, some general comments can be made.

The major sources of air pollution are the combustion of fuels for electricity generation and transportation, industrial processes, heating and cooking. Reactions in the atmosphere among air pollutants may produce a number of important secondary air pollutants, including those responsible for photochemical smog and haze in ambient air.

The spatial distribution and concentrations of the various air pollutants vary considerably. Most air pollutants are a local phenomenon, with concentrations at any particular location varying with local site geography, emission rate and meteorological dispersion factors.

Particulates

Particulate air pollution refers to the presence in air of small solid and liquid particles of various physical dimensions and chemical properties. Although it may be convenient to group them as particulates, their sources, distribution and effects can be highly variable. Some particles can be of natural origin, such as biological particles (pollen, fungal spores, etc), fine soil particles, fine marine salts, wildfire smoke particles and volcanic ash, among other things. Others can originate from a range of sources that include industrial combustion processes, vehicle emissions, domestic heating and cooking, burning of waste crop residues, land clearing and fire control activities. Other fine particulates can be produced in air as a result of slow atmospheric reactions among gases (such as some photochemical smog reactions, or the oxidation of sulphur dioxide and nitrogen dioxide) emitted at distant locations, and transported by atmospheric processes.

The importance of each source varies from place to place, with economic and other conditions. Cities located in low rainfall areas with soils prone to wind erosion may experience periods of high soil particulate levels. In winter, mid-temperate cities of the Northern hemisphere may experience high concentrations of particulates associated with smoke and sulphur dioxide. In summer, many of these cities experience episodes of photochemical smog associated with mixtures of hydrocarbons and nitrogen oxides. Cities in the tropics, particularly those with high vehicle numbers and that are subject to poor dispersion conditions, are prone to episodes of photochemical smog. Cities that are heavily dependent on solid fuels are prone to smoke and sulphur dioxide pollution, particularly those that use coal products for industrial production, electricity generation and domestic heating, such as some cities in Eastern Europe and China. People in rural areas of many developing countries may experience high concentrations of indoor particulate and other air pollution caused by the burning of biomass fuels.

Sulphur oxides

The main sources of sulphur dioxide are the combustion of fossil fuels and industrial refining of sulphur-containing ores. Sulphur dioxide is a colourless gas, which can react catalytically or photochemically with other pollutants or natural components of the atmosphere to produce sulphur trioxide, sulphuric acid and sulphates.

Sulphur dioxide is normally a local pollutant, especially in moist atmospheres, but in oxidized forms it can persist and be transported considerable distances as a fine particulate. It is an important component of acid deposition and haze. Gaseous sulphur dioxide can remain in dry atmospheres for many days and be subject to long range transport processes. As a local pollutant, ambient concentrations of sulphur dioxide may show considerable spatial and temporal variations. Sulphur dioxide concentrations are declining in urban areas of most high income countries, but in many cities of low and middle income countries ambient concentrations continue to increase.

Ozone and other photochemical oxidants

Ozone and other photochemical oxidants are formed in air by the action of sunlight on mixtures of nitrogen oxides and VOCs. A complex series of photochemical reactions produce various oxidants, the most important being ozone and peroxyacetyl nitrate (PAN). Ozone is removed from the atmosphere by reactions with nitric oxide. Ozone concentrations vary with factors associated with the processes of formation, dispersion and removal. Concentrations are higher in the suburbs and in rural areas downwind of large cities than in the city centre, due to ozone removal from the air by reactions with nitric oxide and other components. The concentration of ozone often displays a bell-shaped diurnal pattern, with maximum concentration in the afternoon and minimum concentrations before dawn. Depending on meteorological factors, the highest concentrations occur in summer. PAN concentrations may be 5 to 50 times lower than ozone concentrations, but the ratio can be variable.

PAN concentrations demonstrate the same general diurnal and seasonal patterns as ozone concentrations. Indoor concentrations of ozone are normally substantially lower than outdoor concentrations, although indoor concentrations of PAN may be similar to those outdoors.

Carbon monoxide

Carbon monoxide is a gas produced by the incomplete combustion of carbon-based fuels, and by some industrial and natural processes. The most important outdoor source is emissions from petrol-powered vehicles. It is always present in the ambient air of cities, but it often reaches maximum concentrations near major highways during peak traffic conditions. Indoors it often reaches maximum concentrations near unvented combustion appliances, especially where ventilation is poor. Cigarette smoke contains significant amounts of carbon monoxide.

Nitrogen oxides

Although many chemical forms of nitrogen oxides exist, the most significant from a human health perspective is nitrogen dioxide. The main source of nitrogen oxides in cities is the combustion of fuels by motor vehicles and stationary sources such as industrial facilities. Other industrial processes, such as nitric acid manufacturing facilities, produce nitrogen oxides in air. Urban concentrations tend to be highest near major roads during peak traffic conditions, in the vicinity of major industrial sources and in buildings with unvented sources. Nitrogen oxides are also important indoor air pollutants, as they are produced by domestic and commercial combustion equipment such as stoves, ovens and unflued gas fires. The smoking of cigarettes is an important route of personal exposure.

Lead and other heavy metals

There are several metals regularly found in air that can present real or potential risks to human health. The most important of these are arsenic, cadmium, chromium, lead, manganese, mercury and nickel. On the basis of widespread distribution at concentrations that may damage human health, lead is the most important of these air pollutants on a global basis.

Lead compounds are widely distributed in the atmosphere, mostly due to the combustion of fuels containing alkyl lead additives. As many countries are reducing the lead content of petroleum fuels, or have practically eliminated lead from fuels, this route of exposure is declining. However, high levels of lead in fuels and increasing vehicle numbers are increasing exposure to lead in some countries. Other important sources of lead in air are the mining and processing of ores and other materials containing lead. Inhalation of lead is a significant source of lead in adults, but ingestion of lead in dust and products such as paint containing lead is a more important route of exposure in children.

Arsenic and its compounds are widespread in the environment. They are released into air by industrial sources, including metal smelting and fuel combustion, by the use of some pesticides and, during volcanic eruptions, by wind-blown dusts. Arsenic can reach high concentrations in air and dust near some metal smelters and power stations, mostly as inorganic arsenic in particulate form.

Cadmium is emitted to air from steel plants, waste incineration, zinc production and volcanic emissions. Tobacco also contains cadmium; smoking, therefore, can increase uptake of cadmium.

Chromium is widely present in nature, but it can be introduced into the atmosphere by mining of chromite, production of chromium compounds and wind-blown dusts. It is a component of tobacco smoke.

Manganese is a widely distributed element that occurs entirely as compounds that may enter the atmosphere due to suspension of road dusts, soils and mineral deposits. The smelting of ores, combustion of fossil fuels and emissions from other industrial processes also provide local contributions to the manganese content of the atmosphere.

Mercury enters the atmosphere through natural processes and industrial activities such as the mining and smelting of ores, burning of fossil fuels, smelting of metals, cement manufacture and waste disposal.

Nickel is an element with low natural background concentrations. It enters the atmosphere due to the burning of oils, nickel mining and processing, and municipal waste incineration.

Air toxics

In addition to the well recognized air pollutants, there are many tens of thousands of manufactured chemicals that may be present in indoor and outdoor air. They represent a particular challenge due to the wide variety of chemical types and sources, their widespread prevalence (although often at very low concentrations), the difficulties they present for routine monitoring and regulation, and the time delay for human response. While the effects of acute exposures to these chemicals are easily recognized, the effects of chronic exposures to toxic compounds in air are difficult to detect and it may take decades before they are unequivocally recognized. Toxic compounds present in air may include carcinogens, mutagens and reproductive toxic chemicals (Calabrese and Kenyon, 1991).

There are numerous sources of these chemicals including industrial and manufacturing facilities, sewage treatment plants, municipal waste sites, incinerators and vehicle emissions. In addition to the toxic metals, toxic compounds in air may include organic compounds such as vinyl chloride and benzene emitted by sources such as chemical and plastic manufacturing plants, dioxins emitted by some chemical processes and incinerators, and various semi-volatile organic compounds such as benzo(α)pyrene and other polynuclear aromatic hydrocarbons, polychlorinated biphenyls (PCBs), dioxins and furans emitted by combustion processes.

They may be introduced into the body by inhalation, and accumulate over time, particularly in human fatty tissue and breast milk, although this may depend on the chemical characteristics of the air toxic.

Pollutant mixtures

Most of the work on health responses to exposure to air pollutants has been conducted using single pollutants. Indoor and outdoor air usually contain complex mixtures of air pollutants, and it is practically impossible to examine under controlled conditions all of the combinations of pollutants, exposure concentrations and exposure patterns. In general, mixtures of air pollutants tend to produce effects that are additive (Folinsbee, 1992). Acute responses to mixtures are similar to the sum of the individual responses. The responses to long term exposure to mixtures of air pollutants at chronic exposure levels are unclear.

A summary of the sources of the various major indoor and outdoor air pollutants is provided in Table I.2.

POLICIES AND DEVELOPMENT OF STANDARDS

The premise of this book is that it is preferable to base policy decisions on the best available information, however limited this may be, than to use uncertainty as an excuse for avoiding decisions. Simultaneously, it is important to work efficiently to reduce the uncertainties and provide the basis for more

Table I.2 *Principal pollutants and sources of outdoor and indoor air pollution*

Principal pollutants	Sources
	Predominantly outdoor
Sulphur dioxide and particles	Fuel combustion, smelters
Ozone	Photochemical reactions
Pollens	Trees, grass, weeds, plants
Lead, manganese	Automobiles
Lead, cadmium	Industrial emissions
Volatile organic compounds, polycyclic aromatic hydrocarbons	Petrochemical solvents, vaporization of unburned fuels
	Both indoor and outdoor
Nitrogen oxides and carbon monoxide	Fuel burning
Carbon dioxide	Fuel burning, metabolic activity
Particles	Environmental tobacco smoke, resuspension, condensation of vapours and combustion products
Water vapour	Biologic activity, combustion, evaporation
Volatile organic compounds	Volatilization, fuel burning, paint, metabolic action, pesticides, insecticides, fungicides
Spores	Fungi, moulds
	Predominantly indoor
Radon	Soil, building construction materials, water
Formaldehyde	Insulation, furnishing, environmental tobacco smoke
Asbestos	Fire-retardant, insulation
Ammonia	Cleaning products, metabolic activity
Polycyclic aromatic hydrocarbons, arsenic, nicotine, acrolein	Environmental tobacco smoke
Volatile organic compounds	Adhesives, solvents, cooking, cosmetics
Mercury	Fungicides, paints, spills or breakages of mercury-containing products
Aerosols	Consumer products, house dust
Allergens	House dust, animal dander
Viable organisms	Infections

Source: adapted from WHO, 2000b

informed decisions in the future. This book is intended to support both of these tasks.

Several recent developments make this publication particularly timely. Epidemiological studies in the late 1980s and 1990s, based on time-series analyses, have raised new concerns about some of the most common air pollutants. The results of these studies have been remarkably consistent and have withstood critical examination (Samet et al, 1995; Samet and Jaakkola, 1999; WHO, 2000a, 2000b). The methods used in time-series analyses cannot be expected to prove the possible or probable causal nature of the associations demonstrated between levels of air pollution and health impacts. However, detailed examination of the data and application of the usual tests for likelihood of causality have convinced many experts that the findings need to be seriously considered by policy-makers. The results of the various studies in different cities by different research groups demonstrate associations between air pollutants and health impacts at levels of pollution previously expected to be relatively safe, and below the levels recommended in the 1987 WHO Air Quality Guidelines for Europe (WHO, 1987). Partly as a result, WHO has developed new air pollution guidelines (WHO, 2000a, 2000b).

New insights into air pollution are also providing the basis for new tools for air pollution management. The recent assessments of WHO conclude that for particles and ozone there is no indication of any threshold of effect; that is, there are no safe levels of exposure, but risk of adverse health effects increases with exposure (WHO, 2000a, 2000b). Similar difficulties in identifying a threshold of effect at a population level apply to lead.

This is important for defining air quality guidelines, and indirectly for creating air quality standards. The conventional approach has been to provide a guideline value based on the maximum level of exposure at which the great majority of people, even in sensitive groups, would not be expected to experience any adverse effects. Many users simply interpreted these guidelines' values as if they were recommended standards, which pollution levels should not be allowed to exceed. If there is no such threshold, no single guideline value can be provided by WHO.

To develop standards on the basis of guidelines expressed in terms of unit risks or exposure–response relationships requires explicit decisions on the level of risk considered acceptable. The risk reduction needs to be weighed against the costs and capabilities of achieving proposed standards. Translating this new form of guideline into an air quality standard is superficially more difficult than before. However, guideline values were never meant to be converted into standards, without giving any consideration to prevailing exposure levels or the economic and social context. If applied correctly, the new guidelines should help provide the basis for more appropriate and locally grounded standards (or in some cases the decision to forgo standards).

The relationships upon which the new WHO air quality guidelines are based derive from studies undertaken in affluent countries, and a number of qualifications apply when using the guidelines in low and middle income countries:

1   **The chemical composition of the particles may be substantially different.** The mixture of particles in the communities studied in the development of the particulate guideline was dominated by emissions from motor vehicles, power generation and space heating by natural gas and light oil combustion. The mixtures in communities in developing countries may be different. They may be dominated by different emissions sources with different chemical characteristics, and by wind-blown soil with entirely different toxic properties from those in the studies used by WHO.

2 **The concentration range may be substantially different.** The WHO response–concentration relationships for particulate matter are based on a linear model of response, within the range of particulate concentrations typically found in the studies used by WHO. There are no grounds for simple extrapolation of the concentration–exposure relationship to high levels of particulate pollution. Several studies have shown that the slope of the regression line is reduced when the concentration of particulates is at high concentration levels. These levels may be observed in urban areas in some highly polluted cities in middle income countries.

3 **The responsiveness of the population may be substantially different.** The WHO response–concentration relationships were based on responses of populations that were mostly well nourished and had access to modern health services. By contrast, the populations exposed to higher concentrations of particles in less affluent countries may have a lower level of quality of both nutrition and healthcare. It is not entirely clear whether the responsiveness of the populations in other parts of the world differs from those studies in North America and Europe.

These qualifications imply greater uncertainty in applying the air pollution guidelines in low and middle income countries, but they do not indicate whether the 'true' risks are greater or less than the guidelines assume. From an epidemiological perspective, it may be appropriate to reserve judgement, and to await the results of research designed to test whether similar health effects are evident in communities substantially different from the ones where the original studies were undertaken. A number of such studies are already available and are discussed in this book. In the meantime, however, policy decisions must be made. From a policy perspective, it may be preferable to assume that the same relationships apply, unless there is evidence verifying different relationships. This is the logic that WHO adopted in developing these international guidelines.

Moreover, the degree of caution that ought to be reflected in air pollution standards is itself a policy decision, and one that is usually best addressed through inclusive and consultative processes, which experts and air pollution guidelines can advise but cannot lead. In policy debates, the distinction between risk and uncertainty is often secondary. On the other hand, even the absence of scientific evidence can have a political dimension. Science may be objective in its own terms, but the selection of topics for scientific study is not. The health effects of air pollution have been far more heavily studied in affluent countries largely because of the availability of funds, not because of any prior reason to suspect that health effects are less serious in other parts of the world. Much the same applies to the relatively large amount of attention given to ambient air pollution as compared to indoor air pollution. From a political perspective, there is no overriding reason why the same standard of scientific rigour should be required to motivate policy actions to address comparable problems that have received very different amounts of research. The result would be policies systematically favouring the problems of the affluent.

On the other hand, air pollution standards are only as good as their monitoring and enforcement. There are typically a wide range of measures that can be implemented to reduce air pollution levels and human exposure. These can be grouped according to the pollutants targeted (eg sulphur dioxide, particulates, lead), the pollution sources (eg vehicles, industries, households), the physical means through which pollution is to be reduced (eg improving fuel quality, land use, technologies) or the policy instruments (eg regulation, coregulation, fiscal instruments, tradeable permits, disclosure). It is often possible to identify the major pollution sources and devise targeted measures to reduce their pollution. More comprehensive action requires a systematic approach, with clear policy objectives and regional and other comprehensive plans, including clear allocation of responsibilities, targets, milestones, reviews and continuous improvement initiatives.

Local policy measures are usually inter-related, and it is their combined effect that is important. Vehicular pollution, for example, depends upon land use planning, transport planning, infrastructure investment, traffic management, fuel quality controls and prices, vehicle technology standards and maintenance, and a range of other factors influenced by government policy. Choosing the right combination of measures, and ensuring that they are implemented, is critical. Piecemeal policies can easily work at cross-purposes, incurring high costs to little effect. A coherent strategy, designed in consultation with local stakeholders and supported by an efficient monitoring system, is more likely to reduce air pollution efficiently and yield economic as well as health benefits.

Inevitably, as the causes and sources of air pollution are complex, the matrix of approaches to achieve improvements in air quality requires broad policy mixes, a broad view of regulation and the use of combinations of instruments and actors, and it needs to take advantage of the synergies and complementarities between them (Gunningham and Grabowsky, 1998).

Some important components of an air pollution strategy are listed below, along with examples of the sorts of measures that, depending on the particular setting, can be applied.

An appropriate national policy and regulatory framework. National air pollution standards can be developed to support local air pollution management and resolve inter-jurisdictional air pollution problems. Fuel taxes and subsidies can be designed to reflect contributions to air pollution (recognizing that the impact depends on where the emissions occur). National government can also provide expertise and guidance not available locally, especially in smaller urban centres. And perhaps most important, national governments can help provide local authorities with the fiscal, legal and institutional basis for taking action on air pollution locally.

Local air pollution monitoring. Air pollution monitoring can range from costly systems of air pollution monitors feeding elaborate computer models to low cost systems whose principal role is to identify large changes in pollution concentrations. What is critical is that the monitoring system be designed to support the overall air pollution management strategy.

Public information and health warnings. In cities where air pollution is severe, public information systems can be used to warn local residents of severe pollution episodes, trigger pollution control measures and, perhaps most important in the long run, increase public awareness of air pollution problems. Compulsory public disclosure aims to inform the community about the activities, emissions, discharges and policies of organizations. It relies on the recognition of good performers and the public shaming of poor performers as drivers that improve environmental performance. Examples include the Emergency Planning and Community Right to Know Act in the US. The US Environmental Protection Agency (EPA)'s toxic release inventory is regarded as one of its most efficient and effective instruments. Where pollution is very localized, as in the case of indoor pollution due to the use of biomass fuels, education and awareness programmes can help people take measures to avoid exposure.

Land use planning. A range of tools can be applied to limit urban sprawl and promote mixed land uses, while also ensuring that polluting activities are located in areas least likely to result in human exposure. These tools include land use zoning as well as public infrastructure investment. Since land use planning is typically dominated by other concerns, this requires working closely with government departments for whom public health and environmental protection are not principal responsibilities.

Transport policy. Investments in mass transport systems and making provision for pedestrian and bicycle travel can reduce the use of polluting vehicles. Traffic demand management can reduce congestion in city centres, thereby reducing emissions. Mandatory vehicle inspection and maintenance, retrofits, programmes to remove the most polluting vehicles and emissions standards for new vehicles can also have important effects. Again, this requires working with other government departments while also supporting the overall air pollution strategy.

Industrial pollution abatement measures. Industrial pollution can be addressed directly through emissions standards and obligatory environment and health impact statements, provided that these are backed up by inspections and appropriate enforcement procedures. In some settings, emissions trading systems can be put in place to help ensure that the least cost measures are selected. Where this is not feasible, coregulation and other means of negotiating cost effective improvements are likely to be needed. The promotion of clean technologies, and special programmes for small and medium sized enterprises, can help reduce the costs of reducing emissions.

Energy policy. The reduction of sulphur and organic toxics content and elimination of lead from the relevant petroleum products, taxes on high polluting fuels (eg coal), the introduction of low polluting fuels (eg compressed natural gas and liquefied petroleum gas) and the encouragement of increased use of locally applicable renewable energy can all reduce emissions considerably.

In some cases special measures can be applied in urban centres where emissions are more likely to lead to population exposure. Indoor pollution may also require special measures, but strict regulation is likely to be either ineffective or inequitable, and measures targeted to local circumstances may be needed.

There is enormous variation in the severity and types of air pollution problems experienced in different locations, and their physical, economic, social and political settings. There is no recipe for air pollution management. However, much can learned from the science of air pollution, the various assessment and management tools that have been developed, and the many air pollution initiatives that have been implemented.

SUMMARY OF THE CONTENTS

Following a contextual Chapter 1 that situates the air pollution and health issues in the context of long term development trends and other air pollution problems, the chapters can be roughly divided into three groups:

Chapters 2 and 3: Evidence on the adverse health effects of various types of air pollution. The first of these chapters draws heavily on recent studies in North America and Europe, while the second synthesizes the evidence from studies in developing countries.

Chapters 4, 5 and 6: Tools and approaches to air pollution management. This group includes a chapter describing how international air pollution guidelines and information systems can be used to develop local standards and regulations, a chapter summarizing some of the rapid assessment techniques that can be applied when critical information is lacking, and a chapter on systematic approaches to air quality management.

Chapters 7 and 8: Issues of particular relevance to low and middle income countries. This includes a chapter on the contribution of transport to health-threatening air pollution, and a chapter on indoor air pollution, focusing on the dangers of some highly polluting domestic fuels commonly used in low income countries.

Chapters 9, 10 and 11: Three case studies. The case studies include an analysis of air pollution and the health effects of improvement measures in Hong Kong (China), an analysis of the morbidity and mortality burdens of air pollution in Santiago (Chile) and a broad and holistic view of the policy dimensions of the requirement for air quality improvements in Johannesburg (South Africa).

Although we have tried to ensure as much consistency as possible between the different chapters, their styles reflect the discourses from which they emerge. Thus, for example, the review of recent state-of-the-art studies in the North adopts higher scientific criteria in its selection and presentation of results than the review of existing studies of indoor air pollution in developing countries. Similarly, the more policy-oriented chapters are less questioning of the relation between air pollution and health than the more scientific chapters. In short, the chapters are complementary, but they are not uniform, and are not intended to be.

The health problems caused by air pollution are part of a broader set of environmental problems, and it is helpful to see them in this light. In Chapter 1, Kirk Smith and Sameer Akbar situate the air pollution and health problems of the region in the context of a broader environmental risk transition, wherein the prevailing risks shift from local towards regional and even global scales as one moves from poorer to more affluent settings. They also describe environmental pathway analysis, which provides a common framework for understanding a wide range of environmental impacts, including those on human health. In addition, they examine some of the cross-scale effects, and note some of the trade-offs and opportunities that arise as a result. From this broad overview, it is possible to see how, by paying attention to some of these cross-cutting issues, air pollution damage can be controlled more efficiently.

There is also much of relevance to learn from the current state-of-the-art studies relating air pollution to health. In Chapter 2, Morton Lippmann examines recent evidence from studies undertaken primarily in North America and Europe, focusing on ambient air pollutants. This includes in-depth studies of ubiquitous air pollutants, such as ozone and particulate matter, and their adverse effects on a wide range of documented health indicators, such as mortality rates, hospital admissions, time away from school and work, and lung function. The possible health risks of diesel exhaust are also discussed. Since few of the more advanced studies in North America and Europe have been replicated in low and middle income countries, many health assessments in these countries, including those described in Chapter 6, have drawn on these Northern studies to estimate, for example, dose–response functions for particulates.

In Chapter 3, Isabelle Romieu and Mauricio Hernandez-Avila review the epidemiological evidence on air pollution and health in developing countries, again focusing on ambient air pollution. Several factors, such as nutritional status and population structure, suggest that the adverse health effects may be even greater than those found in developed countries. The data required for the more in-depth studies are not generally available, but the available evidence tends to confirm the view that residents of polluted cities in developing countries are at considerable risk. For example, appreciable risks were found in studies relating to particulate concentrations (PM_{10} – particles with aerodynamic diameters less than $10\mu m$) and mortality in Sao Paulo (Brazil), Santiago (Chile), Mexico City (Mexico) and Bangkok (Thailand). This chapter also reviews the evidence on ozone, nitrogen oxides, carbon monoxide and lead. Clearly, more research is needed in developing countries, but the indications are that the effects of air pollution are at least roughly comparable.

WHO air pollution guidelines have long been important tools for countries developing their own air pollution standards, regulations and policies. In Chapter 4, Dietrich Schwela describes how WHO guidelines can be used to help develop locally appropriate standards, drawing on both local data and modelling and internationally available tools. These guidelines can also be useful for developing the legal framework necessary to translate local standards into effective action. The lack of information can be a significant challenge in many low income cities, however, and additional data collection and analysis are often needed to translate existing guidelines into effective air pollution management systems.

When information is lacking decisions must nevertheless be made, and there are a number of relatively rapid techniques to help support local decision-making. Yasmin von Schirnding describes some of the most important techniques in Chapter 5. Rapid assessments may be needed to respond to a particular event (eg an air pollution episode or a community concern with regard to the pollution from a certain factory), or to help fill in the gaps in the existing information system. Possible techniques range from rapid epidemiological assessments to rapid source-emissions inventories. The mix of techniques required depends upon local circumstances, but it is important that decision-makers be aware of the range of techniques available. To be used most effectively, rapid assessment should not be a one-off effort, but an integral part of the air quality management system.

The importance of taking a systematic approach to ambient air quality management is noted in a number of chapters. In Chapter 6, Steinar Larssen and colleagues describe how a systematic approach can be implemented, drawing on their experience with the World Bank's Urban Air Quality Management (URBAIR) project, which undertook to help create air quality management systems in several cities in low and middle income countries. An air quality management system is an iterative process that can be initiated through the following steps: air quality assessment, environment and health damage assessment, abatement options assessment, cost–benefit of cost-effectiveness analysis, abatement measures selection and design of control strategy. In the participating cities this process helped to identify a number of options whose benefits were estimated to outweigh the costs.

In most low income countries, however, an exclusive focus on ambient air quality is potentially very misleading. As described by Sumeet Saksena and Kirk Smith in Chapter 7, indoor air pollution may be having a large impact on health owing to the use of biofuels, such as fuelwood, to cook (and sometimes heat) in enclosed spaces, especially in rural areas. Among the principal health risks are acute respiratory infection in children, and chronic obstructive lung disease and lung cancer in women. Despite its potentially great importance, most of the research on the health risks of indoor air pollution is recent, with smaller sample sizes and study designs far less sophisticated than those used to study the effects of outdoor air concentrations. In reviewing the results, Saksena and Smith argue that there is emerging evidence that indoor air pollution is associated with important health effects. They describe some of the research needed to understand these effects more fully, and some of the actions that can be taken to reduce the risks.

Turning back to issues of outdoor air quality, Michael Walsh reviews the evidence on vehicle emissions and health in some cities in low and middle income countries in Chapter 8. Vehicles are major contributors to ambient air pollution in many middle income cities, and can lead to particularly high exposures among people situated in heavily trafficked areas. The vehicle fleets of middle income countries are not as large as in many high income countries. However, the popularity of highly polluting motorcycles and scooters, the age and poor maintenance of the vehicles, high usage rates and the continued use of leaded and poor quality fuels lead to high emissions per vehicle for a number of health-damaging pollutants. On the other hand, there have been effective measures to reduce the vehicular pollution in a number of middle income cities and countries. If appropriate lessons are drawn from the successes of existing programmes (some of which are described in this chapter), the relative contribution of vehicles to health-threatening air pollution should decline.

In Chapter 9, Anthony Hedley and colleagues review recent findings in Hong Kong, where air quality is not atypical for a large Asian city. The evidence suggests that the relative risks to health from a number of pollutants are higher than in Western European cities, but that recent control measures have had an appreciable effect on air quality and health. They conclude that policy-makers can be confident that reducing air pollution will provide health benefits, but also note that public concerns over the more visible and easily perceived effects of air pollution have been critical to motivating air pollution control measures.

Chapter 10 addresses one of the first questions local policy-makers and the public typically ask about air pollution: what is the health burden? Bart Ostro provides estimates for Santiago (Chile), a large Latin American city, using a combination of local data and local and international research findings. The results suggest associations between particulate matter and several adverse health outcomes including premature mortality and urgent care visits for respiratory ailments. The findings of these studies are generally similar in magnitude to those reported in other cities in Latin America and throughout the world. As a consequence, it is reasonable to utilize local epidemiological studies and extrapolate the findings from studies in the US.

In Chapter 11, Angela Mathee and Yasmin von Schirnding outline the conditions and processes associated with air quality and health in the city of Johannesburg (South Africa). They review the information gained from studies and surveillance programmes and a number of policies and programmes. They conclude that these studies demonstrate that air quality, especially the high concentrations of particulates in the black urban townships, does not meet international standards and is associated with the high prevalence rates of respiratory symptoms and illnesses in children. Air quality standards based on levels required to protect the most vulnerable in the community need to be introduced and enforced.

Taken together, these chapters raise very serious concerns about the health hazards of air pollution in low and middle income countries, and indicate that much can be done to reduce these concerns. There is, however, a wide range of actors involved, and coordination is of critical importance. There is little point in collecting information if it will not be used, and it is unfortunate when actions are taken on the basis of insufficient information. This is one of the justifications for developing air quality management systems at the local level, and involving all stakeholders in the process. National governments need to provide support for local initiatives, as well as an appropriate regulatory and policy framework. In addition, regional and international cooperation can also make important contributions.

Sharing of experiences and information is an important first step. But in a number of areas, regional cooperation could go beyond this. In research, for example, the problems of indoor air pollution clearly deserve more attention, and in-depth studies – too costly to carry out in every country – could be carried out in a selection of locations. Similarly, there are returns to scale in a number of ambient air quality and health research areas, and joint research initiatives could help overcome the current reliance on studies conducted in European and North American countries where conditions are appreciably different.

Unfortunately, calls for more research are often used to justify inaction. Similarly, calls to action are often used to imply that there is no need for further research. The chapters that follow suggest that both action and research are needed, and indeed that the two should go hand in hand.

REFERENCES

Brimblecombe, P (1987) *The Big Smoke*, Methuen, London

Calabrese, E J and Kenyon, E M (1991) *Air Toxics and Risk Assessment*, Lewis Publishers, Michigan

Elsom, D M (1992) *Atmospheric Pollution: A Global Problem*, Blackwell, Oxford

Folinsbee, L J (1992) 'Human health effects of air pollution' in *Environmental Health Perspectives*, vol 100, pp45–56

Grossman, G M and Krueger, A B (1995) 'Economic growth and the environment' in *Quarterly Journal of Economics*, vol 110, pp353–378

Gunningham, N and Grabowsky, P (1998) *Smart Regulation: Designing Environmental Policy,* Clarendon Press, Oxford

Krzyzanowski, M and Schwela, D (1999) 'Patterns of air pollution in developing countries' in S T Holgate et al (eds) *Air Pollution and Health*, Academic Press, London, pp105–113

Samet, J M, Yeger, S L and Berhane, K (1995) 'The association of mortality and particulate air pollution' in *Particulate Air Pollution and Daily Mortality, Replication and Validation of Selected Studies, The Phase I Report of the Particle Epidemiology Evaluation Project*, Health Effects Institute, Boston

Samet, J M and Jaakkola, J J K (1999) 'The epidemiological approach to investigating outdoor air pollution' in S T Holgate et al (eds) *Air Pollution and Health*, Academic Press, London, pp431–460

Shafik, N T (1995) 'Economic development and environmental quality: an econometric analysis' in *Oxford Economic Papers*, vol 46, pp757–773

Tarr, J A (1996) *The Search for the Ultimate Sink: Urban Pollution in Historical Perspective*, University of Akron Press, Akron, Ohio

UN ECE (1995) *Strategies and Policies for Air Pollution Abatement*, Report ECE/EB, AIR/44, United Nations, New York

UNEP (1991) *Urban Air Pollution*, United Nations Environment Programme, Nairobi

WHO (1987) *Air Quality Guidelines for Europe*, WHO Regional Office for Europe, Copenhagen

WHO (2000a) *Air Quality Guidelines for Europe*, Second Edition, WHO Regional Publications European Series No 91, WHO Regional Office for Europe, Copenhagen

WHO (2000b) *Guidelines for Air Quality*, WHO/SDE/OEH/00.02, World Health Organization, Geneva, http://www.who.int/peh

1

Health-Damaging Air Pollution: A Matter of Scale

Kirk R Smith and Sameer Akbar

ABSTRACT

This chapter presents some key concepts that help to frame the problem of health-damaging air pollution and its relationship with other important categories of air pollution. It discusses the risk transition, which places the shift from traditional to modern sources of pollution along the continuum from household, community and region to the global scale. It describes environmental pathway analysis as applied to health-damaging pollution, focusing on the concept of exposure assessment. Finally, it outlines some of the major cross-scale effects through which pollution problems at one scale relate to problems at other scales, and the trade-offs and opportunities that arise as a result. It concludes that more efficient control of air pollution damage in low and middle income countries today can be achieved with closer attention to some of these cross-cutting issues.

INTRODUCTION

As discussed in the Introduction, public concern about air pollution first clearly manifested itself in the context of ambient air quality in urban areas. Indeed, the first public air pollution commission in recorded history was created in 1285 in London. After deliberating for 21 years, it recommended banning coal burning in urban areas, an action not fully implemented for nearly 700 years (Brimblecombe, 1987). Cities in the rest of the world have also long been paying the social, health and economic costs of elevated levels of air pollution.

In recent decades, however, concerns about urban air pollution have extended to scales previously neglected, including smaller scales such as individual households and larger scales such as entire regions. Accompanying this expansion in scales has been an expansion in the nature of negative health impacts that are of concern.

Examination of air pollution at smaller scales has been necessitated because it has become clear that in some cases potential health impacts are not always well predicted by outdoor measurements. In particular, sources that lead to indoor air pollution may not affect outdoor levels significantly while still resulting in significant ill-health.

Expansion of concern to larger scales has been required because it has become known that some pollutants can travel large distances over time beyond the emission site, thus resulting in regional and global impacts. In some cases, the same pollutant can have different kinds of impacts depending on the scale. For example, sulphur dioxide (SO_2) may have a direct health impact at the community scale and an impact through acid precipitation at a regional scale.

RISK TRANSITION[1]

There is a tendency, although not an inevitability, for peak environmental risks to shift scale from small to large during the economic development process. As shown for South Asia in Figure 1.1, environmental hazards in the poorest communities tend to be dominated by risks related to poor water, food and air quality at the household level. These hazards still dominate the environmental risks for some 1000 million people in South Asia. The spatial and temporal dimensions of such hazards are quite small.

The solutions that are often implemented to address household problems during development (chimneys, drainage, etc) tend to shift environmental problems away from households to the community level, ie smaller to larger scale. They then join with the new types of environmental risks that are created by agricultural modernization, urbanization, industrialization and other aspects of development. About 300 million South Asians live in areas where these risks are likely to dominate.

As these community-scale hazards come under control during further economic development, the most critical impact tends to shift to the regional and global scales through the long term and long distance transport of pollutants. The spatial and temporal scales shift accordingly, as shown in Figure 1.1. In South Asia, as in many other parts of the world, although there are millions of well-to-do people with lifestyles that use energy and resources as intensively as people in rich countries, with consequent impacts on the global environment, their numbers as a fraction of the total population are low.

In much of the world, there are large populations at different levels of development living in close proximity to one another. This creates the potential for environmental risk overlap situations. The principal area of concern in South Asia is indicated by the shading in Figure 1.1, which delineates the region between household and community hazards. In this risk overlap region live approximately 100 million of the urban poor, who simultaneously confront some of the worst household environmental hazards from poor food and indoor air and water quality, and the worst community hazards in the form of

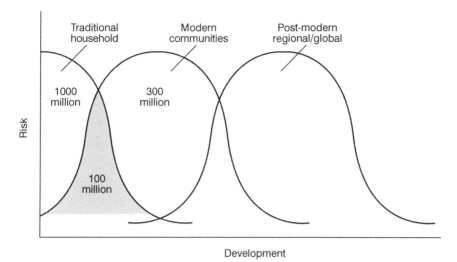

Note: There is a trend in environmental risks during economic development to move from household, to community, to regional and then global scales. The numbers indicate, roughly, how many people are most affected at each scale in South Asia.

Figure 1.1 *Risk transition*

outdoor air pollution, hazardous materials, traffic etc (Smith, 1997). Similar patterns are likely to hold in many other low and middle income regions.

It is generally, although not always, true that economic growth, in addition to extending the temporal and spatial scales of impacts, tends to shift health risks from the direct to the indirect. Direct health risks, for example, result from the inhalation of toxic pollutants. Indirect risks, in contrast, result from processes such as a shift in disease vectors coming from climate change induced by greenhouse gas (GHG) pollutants that may have no direct health impact.

ENVIRONMENTAL PATHWAY ANALYSIS

Illustrated in Figure 1.2 is perhaps the most basic set of relationships in environmental health science: those between sources, emissions, concentrations, exposures and health effects. Although concern with air pollution and other environmental hazards is due to the ill-effects they cause, including to health, waiting until the ill-effects can be reliably determined is not an effective means of controlling the impacts. It is more useful to understand the entire environmental pathway from sources through to health effects. In this way, the most important sources and best points for control can be determined and ill-effects prevented before they occur. The different steps in environmental pathway analysis can be summarized as follows (Smith, 1993):

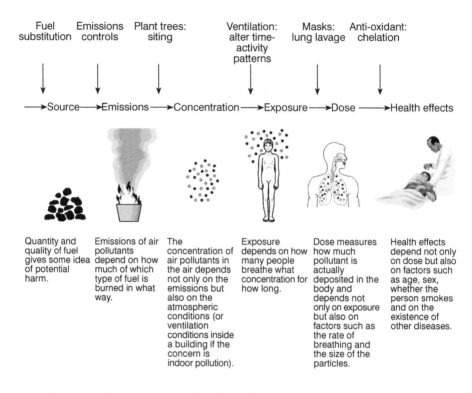

| Fuel substitution | Emissions controls | Plant trees: siting | Ventilation: alter time-activity patterns | Masks: lung lavage | Anti-oxidant: chelation |

$\longrightarrow$ Source $\longrightarrow$ Emissions $\longrightarrow$ Concentration $\longrightarrow$ Exposure $\longrightarrow$ Dose $\longrightarrow$ Health effects

| Quantity and quality of fuel gives some idea of potential harm. | Emissions of air pollutants depend on how much of which type of fuel is burned in what way. | The concentration of air pollutants in the air depends not only on the emissions but also on the atmospheric conditions (or ventilation conditions inside a building if the concern is indoor pollution). | Exposure depends on how many people breathe what concentration for how long. | Dose measures how much pollutant is actually deposited in the body and depends not only on exposure but also on factors such as the rate of breathing and the size of the particles. | Health effects depend not only on dose but also on factors such as age, sex, whether the person smokes and on the existence of other diseases. |

Note: To understand the control pollution effectively it is necessary to understand the entire pathway from source to effect, although measurement and control can occur at any number of places along the pathway.

Figure 1.2 *Environmental pathway*

Step 1: Sources–emissions – Although the type of source (dirty versus clean fuels, for example) gives some idea of hazard, a more valuable measure is the actual amount of pollution emitted.

Step 2: Emissions–concentrations – The most widely used measure, however, is the environmental concentrations of the pollution that results. This depends not only on the emissions but also on the transport, transformation and dilution of the pollutant in the environment.

Step 3: Concentrations–exposures – Environmental concentration, however, is not as reliable an indicator of impact as some measure of exposure. This is the contact of the polluting material with the sensitive system, whether a human, a building or an ecosystem.

Step 4: Exposures–health effects – Not all exposures create the same impact, however, because of differences in the vulnerability of different people or the competing risks that affect them.

Although the pathway in Figure 1.2 refers to ill-health as the endpoint of concern, the same concept can be usefully applied to other important concerns. For example, the endpoint may be ecosystems such as lakes and forests that are vulnerable to acid deposition from regional air pollution. In this case, the important exposures and sources may be entirely different from those that most directly affect health because, among other reasons, the ecosystems are in quite different places than the bulk of the people.[2]

EXPOSURE ASSESSMENT

Most air pollution monitoring and control efforts in low and middle income countries have focused on the emissions and concentrations of pollutants in the outdoor environment (steps 1 and 2 above). In this, they are consistent with the historical development of air pollution management in high income countries. Furthermore, the estimation of health impacts in low and middle income countries has usually been done by extrapolating from concentration/health studies carried out in high income countries to the concentrations measured locally. Unfortunately, this is often the only possible approach because of limited local data.

Data from the region itself should be developed, however, because such extrapolation is subject to question for several reasons:

1   Different exposure levels, ie the average concentrations of concern in many cities in low and middle income countries today are many times greater than the levels studied in most recent urban outdoor studies in high income countries, and there is some evidence of a difference in the effect per unit increase at these higher levels (Lipfert, 1994). Figure 1.3, for example, shows the distribution of urban ambient PM_{10} concentrations in Indian cities containing approximately one-quarter of the national urban population. It should be noted that the mean concentration experienced by the population (194 micrograms per cubic metre, $\mu g/m^3$) is more than six times the US urban mean of approximately $30\mu g/m^3$ (AMIS, 1998).

2   Different populations, ie the pattern of disease and competing risk factors differ dramatically between urban populations in high income countries and people exposed to heavy indoor air pollution in low income countries, who tend to be the poorest and most stressed populations in the world. For example, the overall risk of acute respiratory infections in young children, one of the main impacts of air pollution in low and middle income countries, is many times higher in South Asia and sub-Saharan Africa than in Western Europe and North America, where most air pollution epidemiology has been carried out (Murray and Lopez, 1996).

3   The different relationships between outdoor concentration and actual human exposures because of differences in behaviour, building construction, climate and the prevalence and strength of local sources are not well represented by outdoor monitoring. For example, in tropical climates where housing tends to be well ventilated, in the absence of indoor

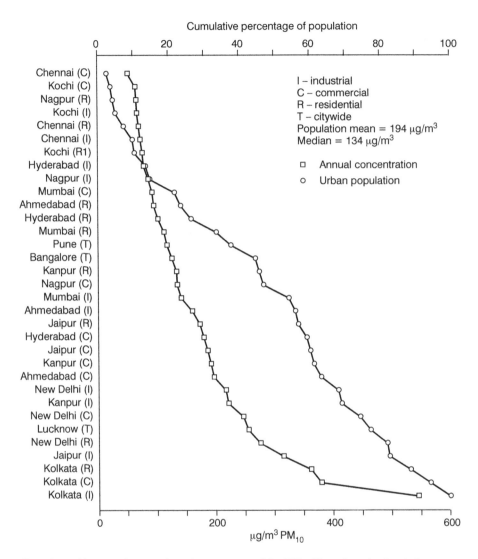

Note: these cities contain approximately one-quarter of the 250 million urban dwellers in the country (AMIS, 1998).

Figure 1.3 *Urban PM$_{10}$ concentrations in Indian cities*

sources, indoor concentrations may be closer to outdoor levels than in temperate countries where most epidemiological studies are carried out. On the other hand, there may be more indoor and neighbourhood sources that are not well reflected in general ambient levels.

4   Different mixtures of pollutants, ie although the concentrations of particulate air pollution of certain size ranges are measured in both cases, the chemical nature of the mixtures may be quite different, for example the higher fractions of diesel exhaust and biomass fuel particles in many cities in low and middle income countries.

These concerns cannot be completely resolved except by studies carried out under local conditions, although as indicated in the following chapters this need not always imply that large scale epidemiological studies, of the sort that have led to a number of recent advances in the understanding of ambient air pollution impacts in Europe and North America, are necessary.

There is in any case a more fundamental problem with the direct application of risk factors derived from outdoor measurements to calculating population impacts – a problem that is also shared in high income countries. To understand the problem it is important to differentiate between the two scales at which typical air pollution health studies operate. Generally, such studies are carried out by examining the way differences in outdoor pollution levels over time or between different populations (cities or parts of cities) correlate with differences in health status in the populations of concern. Thus, the pollution measurements are made at the community level but the health measurements are made at the individual level. In interpreting the results, it is often presumed that the community pollution levels measured accurately represent what individuals experience.

A number of studies carried out around the world, including in low and middle income countries, show that it is often true that the *change* in outdoor levels is reflected in *changes* in the level experienced by individuals. Indeed, this is why so many studies have shown such high correlations between outdoor pollution differences and differences in ill-health. In addition, however, many studies also show that the absolute levels measured outdoors are often quite different from the absolute levels experienced by individuals, because of a combination of less than perfect penetration indoors by outdoor pollutants or local sources (Janssen, 1998; Tsai et al, 2000).

To determine the total health impact of air pollution, therefore, it is preferable to combine the results of the health studies that use exposure information with estimates of the total exposure to the pollutants from other studies designed specifically to take account of where people are in relation to where the pollution is. It may be that the outdoor levels measured in the course of health studies are reliable indicators of total exposure, but it is much more likely that they indicate only part of the exposure – that which is due to outdoor pollutant levels. Indoor or other localized pollutant sources, which may not affect outdoor levels to any degree, can add substantially to total exposures.

Although, once stated, the idea of looking not only at where the pollution is but also at where the people are to determine the total health implications of pollution may seem obvious, it can have a profound impact on how the problem is framed. For example, it alters the relationship between commonly perceived pollution sources, emphasizing how much of their emissions actually reach people's lungs rather than their total emissions. In this way, for example, vehicle emissions, which are released in places and times where people are located, may exert a higher health price per unit of pollution than emissions from large outdoor sources, such as power plants, which release pollutants relatively far from where people reside. It has been shown, for example, that hourly exposure levels for respirable suspended particulate matter on three-wheeler scooters

($782\mu g/m^3$) in Delhi are almost three times the eight-hourly ambient concentration ($275\mu g/m^3$) (Akbar, 1997).

In addition, exposure assessment often also reveals an entirely new landscape of sources and potential control measures. In many low income countries, for example, as discussed in Chapter 7, a large portion of the population's time is spent in homes where solid fuels are burned in open stoves, leading to indoor concentration levels that probably account for a larger total exposure than outdoor sources in the region, even though they do not contribute a majority of total outdoor emissions. This also reveals ways to control exposures that do not rely at all on decreasing outdoor emissions. Indeed, some viable approaches to decreasing exposures, such as disseminating stoves with chimneys, may actually increase outdoor emissions and concentrations.

The concept of exposure is not confined solely to pollutants that produce direct health effects. Examples include pollutants such as nitrogen oxides (NO_x) and sulphur oxides (SO_x), which can produce acid deposition (rain, snow or particles alone) by conversion through atmospheric chemistry, often far from their source, to acidic aerosols (mixtures of liquid and solid particles). Acid deposition is not a problem everywhere. Much of the world's surface is covered with ocean or with soils and vegetation that are little affected by acid deposition. Other areas, however, such as some types of crops, forests and lakes, can be damaged. Whether a certain emission's source creates an exposure of concern, therefore, depends on its orientation and distance from vulnerable ecosystems, local wind patterns, etc. This is exactly parallel to the relationship of health-damaging pollution sources, ie some are much more effective at producing exposure than others.

The same concept applies to GHGs, such as methane and carbon dioxide, which indirectly affect human health through global warming. In this case, the impact per kilogram of emissions can vary dramatically depending on the particular physical properties of the substance and its lifetime in the atmosphere. Over the next 20 years, for example, a kilogram of methane emissions will cause the Earth to be exposed to approximately 60 times more global warming than a kilogram of carbon dioxide. Nitrous oxide, another GHG, is nearly 300 times as powerful as an equal amount of carbon dioxide.

Major Cross-scale Effects

The air pollution implications at each scale are described briefly in the following sections. The discussions rely on the concepts discussed above related to risk transition, environmental pathway and exposure assessment. Briefly, implications are discussed for viable air quality management and ways in which actions at each scale may affect other scales. At the end, some of the trade-offs and opportunities created by the differences are discussed briefly.

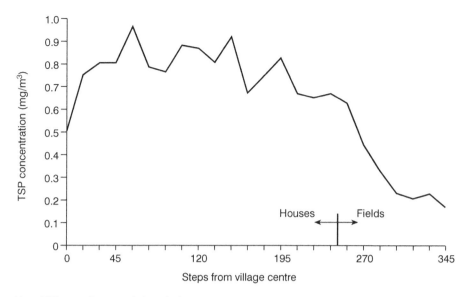

Note: TSP = total suspended particulate matter
Source: Smith, 1987

Figure 1.4 *Neighbourhood pollution in an Indian village in central Gujarat during the winter*

Household/neighbourhood

As discussed in Chapter 7, there seem to be large health implications associated with the uncontrolled combustion of solid fuels in many low income homes due to the resulting household exposures to important pollutants. Efforts to reduce household indoor pollution through the use of chimneys can act to shift the problem to larger scales. In some villages, household pollution can lead to a 'neighbourhood effect', in which outdoor concentrations are elevated in communities with many households using solid fuels. Figure 1.4 shows, for example, outdoor measurements in a village in Western India during the evening meal.

In dense urban areas, household fuels can contribute significantly to general ambient pollution. In addition, however, there can also be significant neighbourhood effects in cities. Figure 1.5 shows results from a study of residential areas in Pune, India. It should be noted that the local outdoor pollution levels in the neighbourhood of biomass-using households are much higher than in gas-using areas, which have outdoor levels similar to the citywide concentrations. Kerosene-using areas seem to be intermediate. It should also be noted that the total exposure of people living in biomass-using households is significantly affected by the pollution coming indoors from outside.

Thus, although improved stoves are sometimes called 'smokeless', they actually still produce substantial pollution. However, when operating well, at least the pollution is vented outdoors. It is clear that such stoves can only be

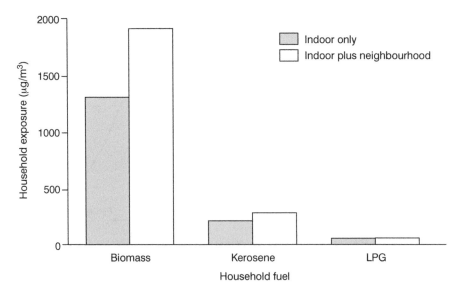

Note: LPG = liquefied petroleum gas
Source: Smith et al, 1994

Figure 1.5 *Urban neighbourhood pollution measured in Pune, India*

considered as an interim solution in such communities. If many people use solid fuels, whether with chimneys or not, total neighbourhood exposures can remain high even for those households not cooking at all or cooking with clean fuels. This situation may also strengthen the argument for programmes designed to convert whole neighbourhoods at once to clean fuels.

Neighbourhood/community

To determine the total exposure to pollutant emissions, it is necessary to consider possible transformations in the environment. Two such transformations act in cities to create pollution outside the local area where the precursor pollutants are emitted:

1   Urban ozone concentrations are a potentially serious threat to health (see Chapters 2 and 3). Ozone is not emitted directly, however, but is formed by a combination of NO_x and hydrocarbon pollutants in the right conditions of temperature and sunlight. Since it takes hours to form, it can be a problem relatively far from the points at which the precursors (nitrogen dioxide (NO_2) and hydrocarbons) are emitted.
2   Particulates are not only emitted directly by fuel combustion and other processes, but are created through chemical reactions in the atmosphere that transform the gaseous pollutants SO_x and NO_x into sulphate and nitrate particles. These particles tend to be more acidic than those directly emitted from fuel combustion and other sources, and some studies indicate that

they may be more toxic by mass than non-acidic particles. Indeed, the new World Health Organization Regional Office for Europe (WHO-EURO) air quality guidelines specify a separate particle-to-health relationship for sulphate for this reason. Ammonia emissions from industry or agriculture can also be converted into particles. As with ozone, all these particles can be formed far from the original emitters, depending on wind, temperature, humidity and other factors.

Community/regional

Particles and ozone can be created outside cities from city sources and impose health risks as well as loss of visibility and damage to crops downwind. In addition, sulphate and nitrate particles can be carried hundreds of kilometres from cities or remotely sited facilities such as power plants to be deposited in dry form or as acid rain/snow (collectively called 'acid deposition'). Such deposition usually imposes little direct health risk, but can damage natural and managed ecosystems with indirect impacts on human health and wellbeing. For example, toxic metals normally bound up in soils may be released and eventually consumed by humans in contaminated fish.

Regional/global

Combustion-generated particles and those created by the downwind transformation of SO_x and NO_x are generally quite small, less than one-millionth of a metre in diameter. Such particles can stay aloft in the atmosphere for months and thus have time to travel around the world. Although the impacts of these particles are not known precisely and are thus the subject of considerable current research, there seem to be two major types of interaction:

1   The particles may form the seeds for clouds, perhaps causing earlier and greater cloud formation than would occur without them, leading to more reflected sunlight.
2   Depending on the character of the Earth's surface below, the particles can be either darker or lighter, thus leading to changes in the amount of reflected sunlight. In general, it is currently thought that the net effect is to reflect more sunlight than would otherwise occur.

The overall effect of global particles is thought at present to have been a net cooling of the Earth, a conclusion supported by the known impact of the suspended dust from large volcanic eruptions. Indeed, emissions of human-generated particles help researchers to understand the discrepancies in the large computer models designed to 'pre-predict' global warming from GHG emissions over this past century. The models generally predict greater warming than has actually been observed, but come much closer to observed changes when the cooling from particles is included.

The message for air pollution control policy seems to be that, as emissions of particles and their precursors come under control because of concerns about

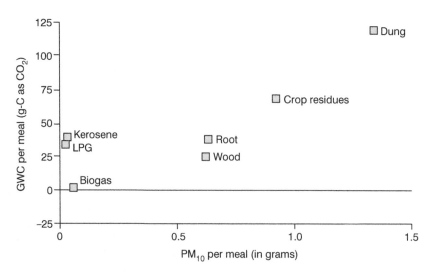

Note: GWC = global warming commitment; g-C = grams of carbon
Source: Smith et al, 1999

Figure 1.6 *Greenhouse gas and PM$_{10}$ emissions from various household fuels illustrating reductions in each that could be attained by fuel switching*

household, community and regional impacts, their capacity to partly shield humanity from the effects of global warming from GHG emissions will diminish.

Household/global

The same incomplete combustion processes in solid fuel stoves that produce most of the health-damaging pollutants (HDP) such as particles, formaldehyde, benzene, etc, also produce important GHGs such as methane. In addition, some of the emitted pollutants, such as carbon monoxide and hydrocarbons, are both HDP and GHG precursors. Typically, 10–20 per cent of the fuel carbon in South Asian solid fuel stoves is diverted to GHGs and HDP, instead of carbon dioxide and water, which would be the products of complete combustion (Smith et al, 2000). Carbon dioxide, of course, is a GHG but, if the biomass fuel is harvested renewably, it does not cause a net greenhouse effect because it is captured during regrowth. Essentially all crop residues and animal dung are harvested renewably, along with a significant, although uncertain, fraction of the woodfuel (Ravindranath and Hall, 1995). However, even renewably harvested biomass fuels have significant GHG potential, because so much of the carbon is diverted to other GHGs, particularly methane, which cause greater warming than carbon dioxide.

As a result, although individually small, household stoves are numerous enough to contribute significantly to the GHG inventories of many low income countries. It is estimated, for example, that Indian household stoves emit about 3 million tons of methane each year, equivalent in global warming to carbon dioxide emissions from the entire transport sector (Mitra and Bhattacharya, 1998; Smith et al, 1999).

The significance of GHGs as well as HDP from household solid fuel combustion may offer an opportunity for influencing GHG control strategies, and ensuring that international funds and agreements devoted to reducing GHG emissions also contribute to improved health (Wang and Smith, 1999). Figure 1.6 illustrates the GHG and HDP benefits that could occur, for example, by a shift from solid to gaseous or liquid fuels in the household sector.

Community/global etc

Shifts in technology and/or fuel in the power, transport and industrial sectors, as well as in the household sector, can result in significant health as well as GHG benefits. It should be noted, however, that there are also shifts in technology that would achieve only one kind of benefit. For example, a shift from natural gas power to hydropower would reduce GHGs with little HDP reduction. A shift from coal to hydro (or gas), however, would achieve both. Thus, to assure a win–win result it is necessary to carefully choose technologies that will achieve both kinds of benefits (Wang and Smith, 1998).

CONCLUDING REMARKS

In low and middle income countries, industrialization, vehicularization and other polluting aspects of modernization are proceeding while many important household and neighbourhood sources still remain important (an example of risk overlap). Since these sources are those in and near households, their actual risks may not be well represented by typical ambient urban monitoring schemes, which have been the focus of developed country control strategies. Thus, to understand the total risk of pollution and the most cost-effective measures available to control its human risk, it is important to consider the exposure implications of different sources, as well as their impacts on urban outdoor pollution levels. Similarly, since pollution can cross boundaries, it is important to consider the relationship between emissions and impacts at household, community, regional and global scales in order to understand the total impact and discover opportunities for efficient control.

NOTES

1   See the discussion in Holdren and Smith, 2000.
2   This simple model needs elaboration, however, when the health impact is the result of an infectious agent, because additional connections must be considered, for example, between infected and uninfected populations.

REFERENCES

Akbar, S (1997) *Particulate Air Pollution and Respiratory Morbidity in Delhi, India*, PhD Thesis, Imperial College of Science, Technology and Medicine, University of London

AMIS (1998) *Healthy Cities Air Management Information System*, Version 2.0, World Health Organization, Geneva

Brimblecombe, P (1987) *The Big Smoke*, Methuen, London

Holdren, J P and Smith, K R et al (2000) 'Energy, the environment and health', Chapter 3 in *World Energy Assessment: Energy and the Challenge of Sustainability*, New York, United Nations

Janssen, N (1998) *Personal Exposure to Airborne Particles*, University of Wageningen, The Netherlands

Lipfert, F W (1994) *Air Pollution and Community Health: A Critical Review and Data Sourcebook*, Van Nostrand Reinhold, New York

Mitra, A P and Bhattacharya, S (1998) *Greenhouse Gas Emissions in India*, Scientific Report No 11, Centre on Global Change, National Physical Laboratory, New Delhi

Murray, C J L and Lopez, A D (1996) *Global Burden of Disease*, Harvard University, Cambridge

Ravindranath, N H and Hall, D O (1995) *Biomass, Energy and Environment: A Developing Country Perspective from India*, Oxford University Press, Oxford

Smith, K R (1987) *Biofuels, Air Pollution and Health*, Plenum, New York

Smith, K R (1993) 'Fuel combustion, air pollution exposure and health: the situation in developing countries' in *Annual Review of Energy and Environment*, vol 18, pp529–566

Smith, K R (1997) 'Development, health and the risk transition' in G Shahi et al (eds) *International Perspectives in Environment, Development, and Health*, Springer, New York, pp51–62

Smith, K R, Apte, M G, Ma, Y, Wathana, W and Kulkarni, A (1994) 'Air pollution and the energy ladder in Asian cities' in *Energy, The International Journal*, vol 19, no 5, pp587–600

Smith, K R, Uma, R, Kishore, V V N, Lata, K, Joshi, V, Zhang, J, Rasmussen, R A and Khalil, M A K (1999) *Greenhouse Gases from Small-scale Combustion in Developing Countries: Household Stoves in India*, USEPA, Research Triangle Park. North Carolina

Smith, K R, Zhang, J, Uma, R, Kishore, V V N, Joshi, V and Khalil, M A K (2000) 'Greenhouse implications of household fuels: an analysis for India' in *Annual Review of Energy and Environment*, vol 25, pp741–763

Tsai, F C, Smith, K R, Vichit-Vadakan, N, Ostro, B D, Chestnut, L G and Kungskulniti, N (2000) 'Indoor/outdoor PM_{10} and $PM_{2.5}$ in Bangkok, Thailand' in *Journal of Exposure Analysis and Environmental Epidemiology*, vol 10, pp15–26

Wang, X and Smith, K R (1998) *Near-Term Health Benefits of Greenhouse Gas Reductions: A Proposed Assessment Method with Application in Two Energy Sectors of China*, WHO EHG/98.12, World Health Organization, Geneva

Wang, X and Smith, K R (1999) 'Near-term benefits of greenhouse gas reductions: health impacts in China' in *Environmental Science and Technology*, vol 33, no 18, pp3056–3061

2

Air Pollution and Health – Studies in the Americas and Europe

Morton Lippmann

ABSTRACT

Studies in the Americas and Europe in recent years on the health effects of ubiquitous air pollutants, such as particulate matter (PM) and ozone (O_3), have documented responses proportionate to exposures, including excess daily and annual mortality, hospital admissions, lost time from school and work and reduced lung function. These effects constitute a significant public health challenge in developed countries where more immediate health and safety challenges are under reasonable degrees of control. Ozone levels in many developing countries are currently lower than in the Americas and Europe, and precautionary controls on sources of hydrocarbons and nitrogen dioxide can be instituted to keep them from rising to levels that produce major effects. Levels of particulate matter in the air in cities in developing countries, especially those due to coal smoke, can be high and the adverse health effects they produce can decrease as emissions are reduced.

INTRODUCTION

Most of the scientific literature on air pollution and human health has been based on studies of populations exposed to mixtures of ambient air pollutants derived from widely distributed combustion sources, and these will be the focus of this paper. There is also an extensive literature on the health effects of air pollutants from specific industrial point sources of toxic and/or cancer-causing chemicals. However, since these are so location- and time-specific and since exposures to populations downwind are so variable, it is not possible to offer any meaningful summary of this literature in the space available. There is a similar difficulty in reviewing the health effects of air pollution derived from indoor sources, especially cooking and space heating with non-vented combustion sources, in terms of the highly variable nature and extent of such pollution over space and time in a given community. This discussion is included in Chapter 7 of this publication.

By contrast, the group of air pollutants known as 'classical air pollutants' by the World Health Organization (WHO) and as 'criteria air pollutants' in the US is attributable to relatively large numbers of relatively small sources throughout a community (space heating and motor vehicles) or to power plants with tall stacks whose effluents are dispersed into the community air. This pollutant group includes some specific primary (directly emitted) gaseous pollutants such as sulphur dioxide (SO_2), nitrogen oxides ((NO_x) emitted primarily as nitric oxide (NO) along with some nitrogen dioxide (NO_2)), and carbon monoxide (CO), as well as lead (in various chemical compounds) as fine particles from the tailpipes of vehicles burning fuel containing organic lead compounds as octane boosters. The primary PM category also includes fine carbon particles from vehicles with diesel engines and coarse particles (with aerodynamic diameters greater than 2.5μm) from soil and soil-like particles resuspended by winds and motor vehicles, or generated by mechanical forces in operations involving agriculture, construction, demolition and various industries.

The classical pollutant group also covers secondary pollutants that are formed in the ambient air by chemical and photochemical reactions of primary pollutants. These reactions include oxidation of NO to NO_2, reactions of hydrocarbon vapours with NO_2 leading to the formation of oxidant radicals and O_3, a highly reactive vapour, and the oxidation of SO_2 and NO_2 to produce ultrafine sulphuric acid aerosol (H_2SO_4) and nitric acid vapour (HNO_3). Further atmospheric reactions of the strong acids with ammonia vapour (NH_3) of biogenic origin, followed by aggregation of the ultrafine sulphate (SO_4) and nitrate (NO_3^-) particles leads to the accumulation of the fine SO_4 and NO_3^- particles that are closely associated with atmospheric haze and acid rain. As secondary pollutants formed continuously and gradually across large geographic areas, O_3 and $PM_{2.5}$ (fine particles with aerodynamic diameters less than 2.5μm) are the most uniformly distributed of the classical pollutants.

Current knowledge about the health effects of the classical air pollutants comes from a variety of sources. The best evidence for SO_2 comes from controlled exposure studies in human volunteers, demonstrating that people with asthma are especially responsive and may have acute respiratory responses (bronchoconstriction) after brief exposures (as low as 0.25 parts per million (ppm)). For CO, the most sensitive members of the population are cardiovascular patients with angina. For such people, controlled exposures that elevate concentrations of carboxyhaemoglobin in the blood to roughly 3 per cent have been found to reduce the time to exercise-induced angina and to cause characteristic changes in their electrocardiograms.

For lead, the clearest evidence for adverse health effects at low levels comes from epidemiological studies, and includes elevated blood pressure in adults and developmental abnormalities in children. For NO_2, there are no clearly established health effects associated with ambient levels, only associations between ambient NO_2 and elevated mortality and morbidity in large population studies. Since NO_2 may simply be serving as a surrogate measure of 'dirty air' in these studies, the jury is still out on a direct role for NO_2.

On the other hand, NO_2 may well be one of the most important of the classical pollutants in relation to the much more substantial effects that have been attributed to exposures to O_3 and $PM_{2.5}$. This is because NO_2 is an essential ingredient (along with hydrocarbon vapours and sunlight) in the photochemical reaction sequences leading to the formation of both O_3 and organic fine particles. Furthermore, the oxidants produced in the photochemical reactions accelerate the transformation of the weak acid vapours (SO_2 and NO_2) into strong acids and their particulate ammonium salts within the $PM_{2.5}$ fraction.

Most of the following in this paper is devoted to a summary review of a broad array of current knowledge on the health effects of the most influential of the classical air pollutants, ie O_3 and fine particles.

HEALTH EFFECTS OF OZONE (O_3)

A great deal is known about some of the health effects of O_3. However, much of what is known relates to transient, apparently reversible effects that follow acute exposures lasting from 5 minutes to 6.6 hours. These effects include respiratory effects (such as changes in lung capacity, flow resistance, epithelial permeability and reactivity to broncho-active challenges). These effects can be observed within the first few hours after the start of the exposure and may persist for many hours or days after the exposure ceases. Repetitive daily exposures over several days or weeks can exacerbate and prolong these transient effects. There has been controversy about the health significance of such effects and whether such effects are sufficiently adverse to serve as a basis for an air quality standard (Lippmann, 1988, 1991, 1993; EPA, 1996a).

Decrements in respiratory function (such as forced vital capacity (FVC) and forced expiratory volume in the first second of a vital capacity manoeuvre (FEV_1)) fall into the category where adversity begins at some specific level of pollutant-associated change. However, there are clear differences of opinion on what the threshold of adversity ought to be. It is known that single O_3 exposures to healthy non-smoking young adults at concentrations in the range of 80–200 parts per billion (ppb) produce a complex array of respiratory effects. These include decreases in respiratory function and athletic performance, and increases in symptoms (airway reactivity, neutrophil content in lung lavage and rate of mucociliary particle clearance) (Lippmann, 1988, 1991). Table 2.1 shows that decreases in respiratory function (mean FEV_1 decrements of greater than 5 per cent) have been seen at 100ppb of O_3 in ambient air for children at summer camps and for adults engaged in outdoor exercise for only 30 minutes.

Further research will be needed to establish the inter-relationships between small transient decreases in lung function, such as FEV_1, peak expiratory flow rate (PEFR) and mucociliary clearance rates – which may not in themselves be adverse effects – and more clinically relevant changes (symptoms, performance, reactivity, permeability and neutrophil counts). The latter may be more closely associated with the accumulation or progression of chronic lung damage.

Table 2.1 *Population-based decrements in respiratory function associated with exposure to ozone in ambient air*

| | Percentage decrement at 120ppb O_3 | | | |
| | Camp children[a] | | Adult exercisers[b] | |
Functional index	Mean	90th percentile	Mean	90th percentile
Forced vital capacity	5	14	5	16
FEV_1	8	19	4	12
FEF25–75[c]	11	33	16	39
PEFR[d]	17	42	13	36

Notes: a = 93 children at Fairview Lake, New Jersey, YMCA summer camp 1984.
b = 30 non-smoking healthy adults at Tuxedo, New York, 1985.
c = Forced expiratory flow rate between 25 per cent and 75 per cent of vital capacity.
d = Peak expiratory flow rate.
Source: Lippmann, 1991

The clearest evidence that current US peak ambient levels of O_3 are closely associated with adverse health effects in human populations comes from epidemiological studies focused on acute responses. The 1997 revision to the US O_3 standard (see Table 2.2) relied heavily (for its quantitative basis) on a study of emergency hospital admissions for asthma in New York City, and its consistency with other time-series studies of hospital admissions for respiratory diseases. However, other acute responses, while less firmly established on quantitative bases, are also occurring. In order to put them in perspective, Dr George Thurston of New York University prepared a graphic presentation showing the extent of related human responses based on the exposure–response relationships established in a variety of published studies. For New York City, as shown in Figure 2.1, a variety of human health responses to ambient ozone exposures could be avoided by full implementation of the 1997 US O_3 standard of 80ppb averaged over eight hours. The extent of effects avoided on a national scale would be much larger (Thurston, 1997).

The plausibility of accelerated ageing of the human lung from chronic O_3 exposure is greatly enhanced by the results of sub-chronic animal exposure studies at near-ambient O_3 concentrations in monkeys (Tyler et al, 1988; Hyde et al, 1989). The monkey exposures related to confined animals with little opportunity for heavy exercise. Thus, humans who are active outdoors during the warmer months may have greater effective O_3 exposures than the test animals. Finally, humans are exposed to O_3 in ambient mixtures. The enhancement of the characteristic O_3 responses by other ambient air constituents has been seen in short term exposure studies in humans and animals. This may also contribute towards the accumulation of chronic lung damage from long term exposures to ambient air containing O_3.

Although the results of epidemiological and autopsy studies are strongly suggestive of serious health effects, they have been found wanting as a basis for standards setting (EPA, 1996a). Scepticism centres on the uncertainty of the exposure characterization of the populations and the lack of control of

Table 2.2 *1997 Revisions: US National Ambient Air Quality Standards (NAAQS)*

I Ozone (revision of NAAQS set in 1979 and reaffirmed in 1993)

	1979 NAAQS	*1997 NAAQS*
Daily concentration limit, ppb	120	80
Averaging time	maximum – 1 hour average	maximum – 8 hour average
Basis for excessive concentration	4th highest over 3-year period	3-year average of 4th highest in each year
Equivalent stringency for 1 hour	maximum in new format, ppb	~90
Number of US counties expected to exceed NAAQS	106	280
Number of people in counties exceeding NAAQS	74×10^6	113×10^6

II Particulate matter (revision of NAAQS set in 1987)

	1987 NAAQS	*1997 NAAQS*	
	PM_{10}	PM_{10}	$PM_{2.5}$
Index pollutant			
Annual average concentration limit, $\mu g/m^3$	50	50	15
Daily concentration limit, $\mu g/m^3$	150	150	65
Basis for excessive daily concentration	4th highest over 3-year period	> 99th percentile average over 3 years	> 98th percentile average over 3 years
Number of US counties expected to exceed NAAQS	41	14	~150
Number of people in counties exceeding NAAQS	29×10^6	$~9 \times 10^6$	$~68 \times 10^6$

confounding factors. Some of these limitations are inherent in large scale epidemiologic studies. Others can be addressed in more carefully focused study protocols. The lack of a more definitive database on the chronic effects of ambient O_3 exposures on humans is a serious failing. The potential impacts of such exposures on public health deserve serious scrutiny and, if they turn out to be substantial, strong corrective action. Further controls on ambient O_3 exposure in developed countries will be extraordinarily expensive and will need to be very well justified. However, precautionary controls on sources of hydrocarbons and NO_2 in developing countries can be instituted to keep them from rising to levels that produce major effects.

HEALTH EFFECTS OF PARTICULATE MATTER (PM)

In Europe and elsewhere in the Eastern hemisphere, particulate pollution has historically been measured as black smoke (BS) in terms of the optical density of stain caused by particles collected on a filter disc. However, it has been expressed in gravimetric terms (micrograms per cubic metre, $\mu g/m^3$) based on

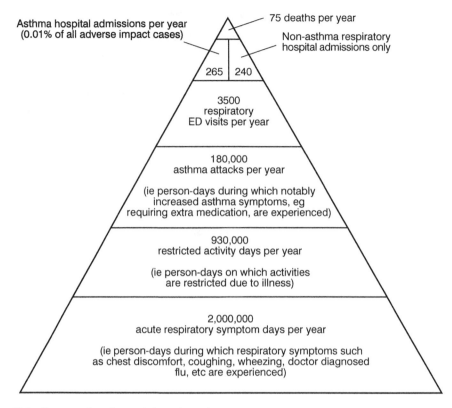

Note: Figure section sizes not drawn to scale.
Source: data assembled by Dr G D Thurston for testimony to US Senate Committee on Public Works

Figure 2.1 *Pyramid summarizing the adverse effects of ambient O_3 in New York City that can be averted by reduction of mid-1990s levels to those meeting the 1997 NAAQS revision*

standardized calibration factors. By contrast, US standards have specified direct gravimetric analyses of filter samples collected by a reference sampler built to match specific physical dimensions or performance criteria.

In the US the initial PM standard, established in 1971, used total suspended particulate matter (TSP) as the index pollutant. The PM standard was revised in 1987, replacing TSP as the index pollutant with PM_{10}. The 1997 US PM standard retained somewhat relaxed PM_{10} limits, but added new annual and 24-hour limits for $PM_{2.5}$, as summarized in Table 2.2.

While justifications for the specific measurement techniques that have been used have generally been based on demonstrated significant quantitative associations between the measured quantity and human mortality, morbidity or lung function differences, established biological mechanisms that could account for these associations are lacking, and there is too little information on the relative toxicities of the myriad specific constituents of airborne PM. In addition to

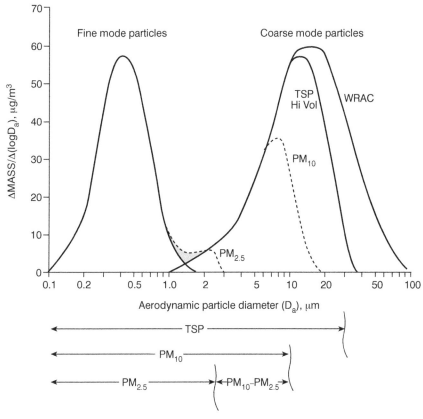

Note: a wide ranging aerosol classifier (WRAC) provides an estimate of the full coarse mode distribution. Inlet restriction of the TSP high volume sampler, the PM_{10} sampler and the $PM_{2.5}$ sampler reduce the integral mass reaching the sampling filter.

Figure 2.2 *Representative example of a mass distribution of ambient PM as a function of aerodynamic particle diameter*

chemical composition, airborne PM also varies in particle size distribution, which affects the number of particles that reach target sites as well as the particle surface area. To date, there are no US standards for the chemical constituents in PM (other than lead) or for the number of particles or surface concentrations of the PM. However, one recent study indicates that the number of fine particles per unit volume of air may correlate better with effects than does the mass of fine particulate matter per unit volume of air (Peters et al, 1997a, 1997b).

A broad variety of processes produce PM in the ambient air, and there is an extensive body of literature that demonstrates that there are statistically significant associations between the concentrations of airborne PM and the rates of mortality and morbidity in human populations. In those studies that reported on associations between health effects and more than one mass concentration, the strength of the association generally improves as one goes from TSP to thoracic particulate matter, such as PM_{10} to $PM_{2.5}$. The influence

Table 2.3 *Comparisons of ambient fine and coarse mode particles*

	Fine mode	Coarse mode
Formed from:	Gases	Large solids/droplets
Formed by:	Chemical reaction; nucleation; condensation; coagulation; evaporation of fog and cloud droplets in which gases have dissolved and reacted	Mechanical disruption (eg crushing, grinding, abrasion of surfaces); evaporation of sprays; suspension of dusts
Composed of:	Sulphate, SO_4^{2-}; nitrate, NO_3^-; ammonium, NH_4^+; hydrogen ion, H^+; elemental carbon; organic compounds (eg polyaromatic hydrocarbons); metals (eg lead, cadmium, vanadium, nickel, copper, zinc, manganese, iron); particle-bound water	Resuspended dusts (eg soil dust, street dust); coal and oil fly ash; metal oxides of crustal elements (silicon, aluminium, titanium, iron); calcium carbonate; sodium chloride, sea salt; pollen, mould spores; plant/animal fragments; tyre wear debris
Solubility:	Largely soluble, hygroscopic and deliquescent	Largely insoluble and non-hygroscopic
Sources:	Combustion of coal, oil, gasoline, diesel, wood; atmospheric transformation products of NO_x, SO_2 and organic compounds including biogenic species (eg terpenes); high temperature processes, smelters, steel mills etc.	Resuspension of industrial dust and soil tracked onto roads; suspension from disturbed soil (eg farming, mining, unpaved roads); biological sources; construction and demolition; coal and oil combustion; ocean spray
Lifetimes:	Days to weeks	Minutes to hours
Travel distance:	100s to 1000s of kilometres	<1 to 10s of kilometres

Source: EPA, 1996b

of a sampling system inlet on the sample mass collected is illustrated in Figure 2.2. The different sampling instruments sample different size groups of PM. This figure also shows that particles have a bimodal distribution in air, with a considerable mass of coarse particles, and fine particles.

The $PM_{2.5}$ distinction, while nominally based on particle size, is in reality a means of measuring the gravimetric concentration of several specific chemically distinctive classes of particles that are emitted into, for example, diesel exhaust, or formed within the ambient air. These include the carbonaceous particles formed during the photochemical reaction sequence that also leads to O_3 formation, as well as the sulphur and nitrogen oxides particles resulting from the oxidation of SO_2 and NO_x vapours released during fuel combustion and their reaction products.

The coarse particle fraction is largely composed of soil and mineral ash that are mechanically dispersed into the air. Both the fine and coarse fractions are chemically complex mixtures. To the extent that they are in equilibrium in the ambient air, it is a dynamic equilibrium in which they enter the air at approximately the same rate as they are removed. In dry weather the concentrations of coarse particles are balanced between dispersion into the air, mixing with air masses and gravitational fallout, while the concentrations of fine particles are determined by rates of formation, rates of chemical transformation and meteorological factors. Concentrations of both fine and coarse PM are effectively depleted by rainout and washout. Further elaboration of these distinctions is provided in Table 2.3.

There is an absence of a detailed understanding of the specific chemical components responsible for the health effects associated with exposures to ambient PM. However, there is a large and consistent body of epidemiological evidence associating ambient air PM with mortality and morbidity that cannot be explained by potential confounders such as other pollutants, aeroallergens or ambient temperature or humidity. Consequently, the US has established standards based solely on mass concentrations within certain prescribed size fractions (see Table 2.2).

As indicated in Table 2.3, fine and coarse particles generally have distinct sources and formation mechanisms, although there may be some overlap. Although some directly emitted particles are found in the fine fraction, particles formed secondarily from gases dominate the fine fraction mass.

The acute mortality risks for PM_{10} are relatively insensitive to the concentrations of SO_2, NO_2, CO and O_3. The results are also coherent, in that the relative risks for respiratory mortality are greater than for total mortality, and the relative risks for the less serious symptoms are higher than those for mortality and hospital admissions.

While there is mounting evidence that short term responses are associated with short term peaks in PM_{10} pollution, the public health implications of this evidence are not yet fully clear. Key questions remain, including:

- Which specific components of the fine particle fraction ($PM_{2.5}$) and coarse particle fraction of PM_{10} are most influential in producing the responses?
- Do the effects of the PM_{10} depend on co-exposure to irritant vapours, such as O_3, SO_2 or NO_x?
- What influences do multiple-day pollution episode exposures have on daily responses and response lags?
- Does long term chronic exposure predispose sensitive individuals being 'harvested' on peak pollution days?
- How much of the excess daily mortality is associated with life-shortening measured in days or weeks versus months, years or decades?

The last question above is a critical one in terms of the public health impact of excess daily mortality. If, in fact, the bulk of the excess daily mortality were due to 'harvesting' of terminally ill people who would have died within a few days, then the public health impact would be much less than if it led to prompt mortality among acutely ill persons who, if they did not die then, would have recovered and lived productive lives for years or decades longer.

Pope et al (1995) linked ambient air pollution data from 151 US metropolitan areas in 1980 with individual risk factors in 552,138 adults who resided in these areas when enrolled in prospective study in 1982. Death records until December 1989 were analysed. Exposure to SO_4 and $PM_{2.5}$ pollution was estimated from national databases. The relationships of air pollution to all-cause, lung cancer and cardiopulmonary mortality were examined using analyses that controlled for smoking, education and other personal risk factors. Adjusted relative risk ratios (and 95 per cent confidence intervals) of all-cause mortality for the most polluted areas compared with the least polluted equalled 1.15 (1.09–1.22) and 1.17 (1.09–1.26) when using SO_4 and $PM_{2.5}$, respectively. Particulate air pollution was associated with cardiopulmonary and lung cancer deaths, but not with deaths due to other causes. The mean life-shortening in this study was between 1.5 and 2 years. The results were similar to those found by Dockery et al (1993) in a prospective cohort study in six US cities, as well as those of previous cross-sectional studies of Ozkaynak and Thurston (1987) and Lave and Seskin (1970). The Pope et al (1995) and Dockery et al (1993) results thus indicate that the concerns raised about the credibility of the earlier results, based on their inability to control for potentially confounding factors such as smoking and socio-economic variables at an individual level, can be eased.

If mean lifespan shortening is of the order of two years, then many individuals in the population have lives shortened by many years, and there is excess mortality associated with fine particle exposure greater than that implied by the cumulative results of the time-series studies of daily mortality. Excess mortality is clearly an adverse effect, and the epidemiological evidence is consistent with a linear non-threshold response for the population as a whole.

HEALTH EFFECTS OF DIESEL ENGINE EXHAUST

Diesel engine exhaust, which contributes a relatively small fraction of the $PM_{2.5}$ in the US and a larger fraction in Europe, has been of special concern because of its odour and its possible effects on cancer rates. In recent years diesel engines have been much more prevalent in light duty applications in Europe than in the US, largely because of the much higher fuel prices. In addition, European concerns for emissions have focused more on global warming than on particles, and diesels emit less CO_2 than equivalent gasoline engines. As a result, the development of light duty diesel engines with performance characteristics acceptable to individual consumers occurred primarily in Europe. Although still called 'diesels', new technology compression ignition engines hardly resemble diesel engines of the past. Tailpipe emissions of soot particles and toxic gases are rapidly approaching the levels of those from gasoline-powered spark ignition engines, while fuel economy and durability continue to increase.

There are concerns for the potential adverse health effects of diesel exhaust because it contains trace amounts of toxic compounds and because occupational exposures are common and environmental exposures are widespread. Diesel exhaust is a ubiquitous component of air pollution. All populations living in developed countries are exposed frequently to diesel exhaust at some concentration. While the potential for diesel exhaust to present a health hazard has been known for several decades, the current emphasis dates to the late 1970s when extracts from diesel soot were found to be mutagenic to bacteria. Research during the last 20 years focused on the potential contribution of diesel exhaust to human lung cancer risk.

Concern for the cancer risk of diesel exhaust has centred on the organic hydrocarbons associated with soot particles. Soot consists of aggregates of spherical primary particles that form in the combustion chamber, grow by agglomeration and are emitted as clusters having average particle diameters ranging from 0.1 to 0.5µm (Cheng et al, 1984). As released to the environment, the portion of the mass of diesel soot consisting of adsorbed organic matter can range from 5–90 per cent (Johnson, 1988). Values of 10–15 per cent are representative of modern engines under most operating conditions. The size of diesel soot particles makes it readily respirable. Approximately 20–30 per cent of the inhaled particles in diluted exhaust would be expected to deposit in the lungs and airways of humans (Snipes, 1989).

The partitioning of compounds between the gas and particulate phases of exhaust depends on the vapour pressure, temperature and concentration of each chemical in the exhaust. Although the potential effects of hydrocarbon vapours are not well understood, little concern has been raised for the long term health effects of these compounds. Lung tumours are not induced in rats by chronic exposure to high concentrations of diesel exhaust if the exhaust is filtered and animals are exposed to only the gas and vapour phases.

The volatile compounds in diesel exhausts are not without adverse effects. People exposed to high concentrations of diesel exhaust complain about objectionable odour, headache, nausea and eye irritation, symptoms thought to be primarily associated with the gas and vapour phase constituents. It is not known if there is any link between these transient symptoms and other health effects. The US Environmental Protection Agency (EPA) estimated that the US annual average concentration of airborne diesel soot in 1990 was 1.8µg/m^3, and that the urban and rural averages were 2.0 and 1.1µg/m^3 respectively (EPA, 1993). The urban, rural and nationwide average concentrations were predicted to fall to 0.4, 0.2 and 0.4µg/m^3 respectively by 2010.

The most relevant information on the human health risks from exposures to potential toxicants is obtained from studies of humans, assuming that the information is adequate for establishing exposure–effects relationships. Numerous epidemiological studies of the relationship between diesel exhaust exposure and lung cancer have been reported, with some studies focusing specifically on diesel exhaust and others on occupations receiving substantial diesel exhaust exposures. This body of information, while large, is weakened by the lack of direct measures of the exhaust exposures of the populations studied. The weight of the epidemiological evidence suggests a positive effect of small magnitude, but confidence in conclusions drawn from this largely circumstantial evidence is eroded by uncertainties regarding exposure and potential confounding by cigarette smoking and other exposures. Contemporary reviews of this information have been published by EPA (1994), HEI (1995) and California EPA (1997).

In the absence of definitive data from humans, hazard characterization and risk assessment typically use data from animals exposed experimentally to the agent in question. Regarding the carcinogenicity of diesel exhaust, however, results from animals have not proved to be very helpful because essentially the same lung tumour response is obtained with pure carbon soot and other inert particles as with diesel exhaust at comparable mass concentrations (Mauderly, 2000).

While it is plausible that diesel soot presents a carcinogenic hazard, there is little consensus of opinion regarding the existence or magnitude of lung cancer risk under current occupational or environmental exposure conditions. The aggregate epidemiological data suggest that occupational exposures may slightly increase lung cancer risk, but do not provide a basis for quantitative estimates of risk with confidence. Overall, it is reasonable to assume that, if the inhalation of airborne mutagenic material is attended by cancer risk, then environmental diesel soot contributes in some measure to that pool of material and thus to the risk. It is also reasonable to assume that cancer risk might parallel the deposited dose of inhaled mutagenic material, depending on the bio-availability of the material and its mutagenic potency in humans.

DISCUSSION AND CONCLUSIONS

Air pollutants can adversely affect human health in a number of ways, both directly and indirectly. Direct effects in downwind populations can range from acute intoxication and prompt mortality from peak point source discharges, as in the Bhopal, India methyl isocyanate release, to delayed developmental deficits resulting from chronic lead exposure in people living near the Port Pirie lead smelter in South Australia. Indirect effects can include those resulting from a primary pollutant such as NO_2 from combustion sources being essential to O_3 formation in the atmosphere, with O_3 having the largest impact on the health effects that result. Indirect effects can also result from acidic sulphur and nitrogen compounds that deposit on soil and leach toxic metals from the soil that bio-accumulate in food crops and flesh that are ingested. Such diverse and complex aspects of air pollution and health are too broad for discussion in this paper. Rather, this review has been limited to the effects of the most ubiquitous air pollutants in both developed and developing countries that are attributable to transportation and space heating sources, ie O_3, PM and diesel engine exhaust.

O_3, resulting from atmospheric chemical reactions involving hydrocarbon vapours, nitrogen dioxide (NO_2) and sunlight, causes reduced lung function, airway inflammation, increased usage of physicians and hospitals, and lost time from school and work following exposures that frequently occur in major urban areas of North and South America. Concentrations of O_3 in many developing countries are lower at the present time, but can be expected to rise in proportion to increasing motor vehicle use. This is further discussed in the following chapter, and in Chapter 8.

The concentrations of thoracic particulate matter (PM_{10}) and fine particulate matter ($PM_{2.5}$) in ambient air are significantly associated with excess daily mortality, annual mortality and daily hospital admissions for respiratory and cardiovascular causes, as well as increased rates of bronchitis in children, lost time from work and school and reduced lung function following exposures at current levels in the Americas and Western Europe. Concentrations of PM_{10} and $PM_{2.5}$ are much higher in cities of many developing countries than they are in the US or Europe, and studies of mortality rates and lung function in some developing countries have produced coherent findings. There is no evidence for a threshold in any of the PM-associated health effects and it is therefore reasonable to expect that reductions in PM exposures in developing countries will result in proportionate reductions in the health effects associated with PM, as discussed in the following chapter.

The concentrations of diesel exhaust are much more spatially variable than those of O_3 or PM, and their odour and nuisance effects, as well as their potential for producing lung cancer, will be much greater for those living or working near major roadways than for people further away. At this point in time, strategies to reduce diesel exhaust pollution should be incorporated into overall strategies to reduce PM pollution.

ACKNOWLEDGEMENTS

This research was undertaken, in part, by the author as part of a programme supported by Grant ES 00260 from the National Institute of Environmental Health Sciences. It has also been based, in part, on material contained in the chapters on ambient particulate matter and ozone written by the author and on the chapter on diesel exhaust written by Dr Joe L Mauderly for the second edition of M Lippmann (ed), *Environmental Toxicants–Human Exposures and Their Health Effects*, published by Wiley in 2000.

REFERENCES

California EPA (Environmental Protection Agency) (1997) *Health Risk Assessment for Diesel Exhaust*, Office of Environmental Health Hazard Assessment, Sacramento

Cheng, Y S, Yeh, H C, Mauderly, J L and Mokler, B V (1984) 'Characterization of diesel exhaust in a chronic inhalation study' in *American Industrial Hygiene Association Journal*, vol 45, pp547–555

Dockery, D W, Pope, C A III, Xu, X, Spengler, J D, Ware, J H, Fay, M E, Ferris, B G Jr and Speizer, F E (1993) 'An association between air pollution and mortality in six US cities' in *New England Journal of Medicine*, vol 329, pp1753–1759

EPA (US Environmental Protection Agency) (1993) *Motor Vehicle-Related Air Toxics Study*, EPA 420–R–93–005, Office of Mobile Sources, Emission Planning and Strategies Division, Ann Arbor, MI

EPA (US Environmental Protection Agency) (1994) *Health Assessment Document for Diesel Emissions*, Volumes I and II, EPA/600/8–90/057Ba, Office of Research and Development, Washington, DC

EPA (US Environmental Protection Agency) (1996a) *Air Quality Criteria for Ozone and Related Photochemical Oxidants*, EPA/600/P–93/004F, National Center for Environmental Assessment, Research Triangle Park, NC

EPA (US Environmental Protection Agency) (1996b) *Air Quality Criteria for Particulate Matter*, EPA/600/P–95/001F, National Center for Environmental Assessment, Research Triangle Park, NC

HEI (Health Effects Institute) (1995) *Diesel Exhaust: A Critical Analysis of Emissions, Exposure, and Health Effects*, A Special Report of the Institute's Diesel Working Group, Health Effects Institute, Cambridge, MD

Hyde, D M, Plopper, C G, Harkema, J R, St George, J A, Tyler, W S and Dungworth, D L (1989) 'Ozone-induced structural changes in monkey respiratory system' in T Schneider et al (eds) *Atmospheric Ozone Research and Its Policy Implications*, Elsevier, Nijmegen, The Netherlands, pp525–532

Johnson, J H (1988) 'Automotive emissions' in A Y Watson et al (eds) *Air Pollution, The Automobile, and Public*, National Academy Press, Washington, DC, pp39–75

Lave, L B and Seskin, E P (1970) 'Air pollution and human health' in *Science,* vol 169, pp723–733

Lippmann, M (1988) 'Health significance of pulmonary function responses to airborne irritants' in *Journal of the Air Pollution Control Association,* vol 38, pp881–887

Lippmann, M (1991) 'Health effects of tropospheric ozone' in *Environmental Science and Technology*, vol 25, no 12, pp1954–1962

Lippmann, M (1993) 'Health effects of tropospheric ozone: implications of recent research findings to ambient air quality standards' in *Journal of Exposure Analysis and Environmental Epidemiology*, vol 3, pp103–129

Mauderly, J L (2000) 'Diesel exhaust' in M Lippmann (ed) *Toxicants: Human Exposures and Their Health Effects*, 2nd Ed, Wiley, New York

Ozkaynak, H and Thurston, G D (1987) 'Associations between 1980 US mortality rates and alternative measures of airborne particle concentration' in *Risk Analysis*, vol 7, pp449–461

Peters, A, Wichmann, H E, Tuch, T, Heinrich, J and Heyder, J (1997a) 'Respiratory effects are associated with the number of ultrafine particles' in *American Journal of Respiratory and Critical Care Medicine*, vol 155, pp1376–1383

Peters, A, Döring, A, Wichmann, H E and Koenig, W (1997b) 'Increased plasma viscosity during an air pollution episode: a link to mortality?' in *Lancet*, vol 349, pp1582–1587

Pope, C A III, Thun, M J, Namboodiri, M, Dockery, D W, Evans, J S, Speizer, F E and Heath, C W Jr (1995) 'Particulate air pollution is a predictor of mortality in a prospective study of US adults' in *American Journal of Respiratory and Critical Care Medicine*, vol 151, pp669–674

Snipes, M B (1989) 'Long-term retention and clearance of particles inhaled by mammalian species' in *Critical Reviews in Toxicology*, vol 20, pp175–211

Thurston, G D (1997) Testimony submitted to US Senate Committee on Environment and Public Works, Subcommittee on Clean Air, Wetlands, Private Property, and Nuclear Safety

Tyler, W S, Tyler, N K, Last, J A, Gillespie, M J and Barstow, T J (1988) 'Comparison of daily and seasonal exposures of young monkeys to ozone' in *Toxicology*, vol 50, pp131–144

3

Air Pollution and Health in Developing Countries: A Review of Epidemiological Evidence

Isabelle Romieu and Mauricio Hernandez-Avila

ABSTRACT

A review of evidence from developed nations substantiates the harmful effects of air pollutants on health, even at levels considerably lower than those observed in many megacities of the developed world. Differences in relation to the level of exposure and co-exposure to different pollutant mixtures, the population structure, the nutritional status and the lifestyle observed in developing nations suggest that the adverse effects of air pollution may be even greater than those observed in developed nations. In this chapter, the epidemiological studies that describe the health effects of various air pollutants (including particulate matter, sulphur dioxide, nitrogen dioxide, ozone, carbon monoxide and lead) are reviewed for different cities of the developing world. Reports from developing nations show similar effects observed throughout the world, adding support for a causal relationship between air pollution and health effects. Various studies have documented increased mortality, visits for respiratory emergencies, higher frequencies of respiratory symptoms and low pulmonary function associated with particulate pollution (particularly with particulates smaller than 2.5 microns ($PM_{2.5}$)). Young children appear to be at higher risk for acute respiratory infections leading to increased mortality and morbidity. Time-series studies evaluating associations between ozone and daily mortality have been inconsistent; however, studies on the health effects of ozone have documented increases in emergency visits and hospital admissions due to respiratory diseases, increases in respiratory symptoms and temporary lung function impairments. Asthmatic populations appear to be more susceptible to the impact of particulate, sulphur dioxide and ozone exposure. Few studies have been reported for carbon monoxide; however, limited data suggest that carbon monoxide exposure is prevalent and may be associated with prematurity and *intra-uterine death. Recent trends indicate that lead exposure is decreasing due to changes in gasoline formulation. However, other sources remain uncontrolled and health effects in cognitive development have been reported. Because complex pollution mixtures are present in the urban areas where most epidemiological studies were conducted, the specific effects and levels at which each pollutant will affect health cannot be readily determined. Chronic exposure is of major concern in developing nations given the high levels of air pollutants observed all year long, but few data are available. Susceptible groups, such as young children, may be at greater risk for adverse health effects given the generally poor environmental conditions and nutritional status that are highly prevalent in developing nations.*

INTRODUCTION

Concern about the health effects of the high levels of air pollution observed in many megacities of the developing world is growing; moreover, it is likely that this problem will continue to grow because developing countries are trapped in the trade-offs of economic growth and environmental protection. There is an urgent need for the implementation of control programmes to reduce levels of pollutant emissions. To be effective, these programmes should include the participation of the different stakeholders and initiate activities to identify and characterize air pollution problems, and to estimate potential health impacts. The impact of each pollutant on human health has proved difficult to establish; questions regarding which pollutant to target and how to reduce exposure should consider local conditions and should be a matter for careful discussion given the high cost associated with environmental interventions.

In many developing countries economic growth without adequate environmental protection has resulted in widespread environmental damage, creating new environmental problems. Populations in urban areas are at risk of suffering adverse health effects due to rising problems of severe air and water pollution.

Although air pollution is recognized as an emerging public health problem, most developing nations do not have data to evaluate its real dimension. The fact that air pollution coexists with other important public health problems, such as low immunization coverage, malnutrition or sanitation deficiencies – which are given higher priority in circumstances where economical resources are scarce – has delayed the actions needed to adequately assess, evaluate and control air pollution in most urban conglomerates in the developing world.

The health effects of air pollution have been thoroughly studied in developed nations (see Chapter 2). A review of the current evidence substantiates the harmful effects of air pollutants, even at levels considerably lower than those commonly registered in many cities in the developed world (Lippmann, 1993; American Thoracic Society, 1996; EPA, 1996, Thurston and Ito, 1999; Pope and Dockery, 1999; Cohen and Nikula, 1999; Pope, 2000). Although air pollutants are likely to have similar adverse effects on different human populations, the range of exposure, co-exposure to different pollutant mixtures, the population structure, the nutritional status and the lifestyle observed in developing nations suggest that the potential health effects of air pollution may be even greater than those reported for developed nations. In this chapter, the epidemiological studies describing health effects of air pollution in developing nations are reviewed briefly. This review was restricted to studies that have evaluated health effects in relation to exposure to the critical air pollutants (particulate matter, sulphur dioxide, nitrogen dioxide, ozone, carbon monoxide and lead), due to the fact that information regarding atmospheric levels of these pollutants is becoming available for major cities in the developing world (Romieu et al, 1990; WHO, 1997). Other air pollutants, such as volatile organic compounds, have adverse health effects, but little is known about their ambient levels in developing countries.

GLOBAL CONCENTRATION PATTERNS OF OUTDOOR AIR POLLUTION

During the past 25 years, the commonly measured indicators of urban air quality have tended to improve throughout the industrialized world (Holdren and Smith, 2000). In contrast, in many developing countries the rapid growth of urban population, the development of industry, the intensification of traffic with limited access to clean fuel and the lack of effective control programmes have led to high levels of air pollution. The Air Management Information System (AMIS) of the World Health Organization (WHO, 1997) provides comparative data on major air pollutant levels across cities in more than 60 countries. Figure 3.1 represents the annual mean and annual change of respirable particulate matter (PM_{10}) concentrations in residential areas of cities in developing countries.

During the 1990s, an increasing trend in PM_{10} concentrations was observed in Asian cities, while in large cities of Latin America, small decrements of PM_{10} concentrations were observed (Figure 3.1). In most cities of developing countries, the annual mean concentration of sulphur dioxide in residential areas did not exceed 50 micrograms per cubic metre ($\mu g/m^3$) with the exception of some cities in China and Nepal, where elevated levels were mostly related to the combustion of sulphur-containing coal for domestic use. The annual mean concentrations of nitrogen dioxide remained moderate, that is, not exceeding $40\mu g/m^3$ in most cities. However, in cities that have both a high volume of vehicular emission and intensive ultraviolet (UV) radiation, photochemical reactions involving NO_2 and hydrocarbons result in high ozone levels. For example, ozone concentrations in Mexico City exceeded the WHO air quality guidelines ($120\mu g/m^3$ over an eight-hour average) on more than 300 days in 1997 (Krzyzanowski and Schwela, 1999; Lacasaña et al, 1999).

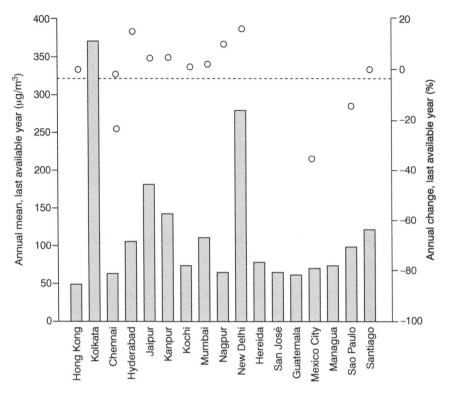

Note: Annual change is given as a percentage of the last available year mean.
Source: Krzyzanowski and Schwela, 1999

Figure 3.1 *Annual mean in last available year (bars) and annual change of respirable particulate matter (PM$_{10}$) concentrations (*) in residential areas of cities in developing countries*

HEALTH EFFECTS OF PARTICULATE MATTER AND SULPHUR DIOXIDE (SO$_2$)

Particulates and sulphur dioxide (SO$_2$) can result from the combustion of fossil fuel. Depending on the source, the ratio of particulates to SO$_2$ in the ambient air may vary (American Thoracic Society, 1996). In areas where fossil fuels with a high sulphur content are used, such as in Beijing, China, high levels of SO$_2$ may be reached, especially during the warm season.

Particulate matter is a product of many processes: soil erosion, road dust, forest fires, land-clearing fires and agricultural burning (American Thoracic Society, 1996). Particulates range over several categories of magnitude in size and, as discussed in Chapter 2, particulate material of less than 10 microns in size may be inhaled into the respiratory system resulting in adverse health effects. Acute exposure to inhalable particulates can result in loss of lung function, onset of respiratory symptoms, aggravation of existing respiratory conditions and increased susceptibility to infection. These problems may occur to a greater degree in asthmatics, small children and the elderly with chronic respiratory and cardiovascular diseases (American Thoracic Society, 1996; Pope and Dockery, 1999; Pope, 2000).

Current concerns about the health effects of airborne particles are largely based on results of recent epidemiological studies. These suggest an increase in mortality and morbidity at levels below the current standards, and a stronger (roughly twice that previously reported) and more consistent effect of fine particles (smaller than 2.5µm) that appear to contain more of the reactive substance potentially linked to health effects (EPA, 1996; Schwartz, 1996; Klemm, 2000; Pope, 2000). Particulate matter is one of the major air pollutants in developing countries where levels frequently exceed current guidelines to protect health (HEI, 1988; WHO, 1993; WHO, 1997).

There is no clear known biological mechanism by which particulate air pollution could affect human health. Increased rates of sudden death, arrhythmic complications and increased plasma viscosity, and reduced heart rate variability have all been described in relation to ambient concentrations of fine particulate matter. In addition, particulate air pollution derived from fossil fuel burning has been shown to impair inflammatory and host defence functions of the lung (Thomas and Zelikoff, 1999). Studies of changes in host susceptibility in response to diesel engine emissions have also suggested that exposures to diesel engine emissions can increase the severity of influenza virus infection and that effects may be mediated by induced changes in interferon (Thomas and Zelikoff, 1999).

Premature mortality

Acute exposure

There is an extensive body of literature on the impact of particulates on mortality. Recent studies relating to the occurrence of daily deaths (total deaths and subdivided by cause) to daily changes in air pollution levels have provided strong evidence of the health effects associated with particulate pollution (Dockery and Pope, 1996; Pope and Dockery, 1999; Pope, 2000). Recently a study summarizing data from 20 cities in the US, reported an increase in total mortality of 0.51 per cent (95 per cent confidence interval (CI) 0.07–0.93 per cent) per $10µg/m^3$ of PM_{10}. For cardiovascular mortality, this estimate reached 0.68 per cent (95 per cent CI 0.20–1.16) (Samet et al, 2000). In addition, the relationship appears to be linear down to the lowest levels where there is no threshold (Schwartz and Zanobetti, 2000), and to affect subjects who otherwise could have survived for a substantial amount of time (Zeger et al, 1999). Daily mortality appears to be more strongly associated with concentrations of $PM_{2.5}$ than with concentrations of larger particles (Schwartz et al, 1996; Klemm et al, 2000). This has special implications for developing countries where vehicular traffic with poorly maintained engines and extensive use of diesel fuel is a major source of particulate pollution.

Mortality studies conducted in developing countries are consistent with estimates from the US and Europe (Borja-Aburto et al, 1997; Hong et al, 1999;

Tellez Rojo et al, 2000; Cifuentes et al, 2000). A major concern has been raised recently concerning the increased infant mortality linked to particulate exposure in Brazil, Mexico and Thailand (Loomis et al, 1999; Ostro et al, 1999; Gouveia et al, 2000; Conceiao et al, 2001). A summary estimate of these time-series studies suggests that an increase of $10\mu g/m^3$ of PM_{10} could be associated with an increase close to 1 per cent in total mortality for respiratory causes in children less than five years of age (Romieu, personal communication).

Chronic exposure

Long term exposure to air pollutants is a major concern for developing countries given that in the majority of cities, the population is chronically exposed to particulate levels exceeding current guidelines to protect health. Two cohort studies conducted in the US have reported a large mortality estimate related to long term exposure to fine particulates. These estimates suggested an increase in mortality from 17 per cent to 26 per cent over a range of approximately $20\mu g/m^3$ of $PM_{2.5}$ (Dockery et al, 1993; Pope et al, 1995). In addition, post-neonatal mortality has been associated with exposure to PM_{10} during the first two months of life. An increase of 25 per cent in overall post-neonatal mortality was observed for $30\mu g/m^3$ range of PM_{10} concentrations (Woodruff et al, 1997). Currently there are no data available from developing countries on the effects of long term exposure to air pollutants on mortality.

Morbidity

Acute exposure

Most of the studies on emergency visits and hospital admissions for respiratory or cardiovascular illnesses conducted in Western countries have reported an increase of 1 to 3 per cent in relation to a $10mg/m^3$ increase in PM_{10}, on the day of the visit or one to two days before the visit (Pope and Dockery, 1999; Pope, 1999). Studies conducted in developing countries to determine the impact of particulate pollution on respiratory emergencies and medical visits have also suggested that increases in air pollution are associated with an increase in the frequency of visits to medical services (Table 3.1).

Studies related to the evaluation of respiratory health in general have observed a higher frequency of respiratory symptoms and lower pulmonary functions in subjects exposed to particulates from combustion sources. Asthmatics appear to be more susceptible to the impact of particulate and SO_2 exposure, and an increase in respiratory symptoms and a decrease in lung function related to exposure to PM_{10} have been documented (American Thoracic Society, 1996; Pope and Dockery, 1999). In addition, diesel particulate has been shown to increase allergic response and might be a risk factor for the development of allergy and asthma (Diaz-Sanchez et al, 1999).

Particulate air pollution may also play a major role in the incidence of acute respiratory infection in children. Various studies conducted in Brazil, Chile, Cuba and Mexico have shown an increased risk of respiratory infections in young children exposed to particulate pollution (Tellez-Rojo et al, 1997; Pino et

Table 3.1 *Health outcomes associated with changes in daily mean ambient levels of particulate (PM concentrations in $\mu g/m^3$)*

Health effects indicators	$PM_{2.5}$	PM_{10}
Daily mortality (children <5)		
Total mortality		
Change of 5%	–	35[a]
Change of 10%	–	65
Change of 20%	–	130
Daily mortality (65 years and over)		
Total mortality		
Change of 5%	–	50[b]
Change of 10%	–	100
Change of 20%	–	200
Respiratory mortality		
Change of 5%	–	25[b]
Change of 10%	–	50
Change of 20%	–	100
Daily respiratory morbidity (Emergency visits for respiratory causes among children)		
Change of 5%	40[c]	80[c]
Change of 10%	80	160
Pneumonia		
Change of 5%	10	20
Change of 10%	20	40
Exacerbation of respiratory symptoms in children with moderate asthma		
Change of 5%	–	10[d]
Change of 10%	–	20
Change of 20%	–	20
Peak expiratory flow rate in children with moderate asthma		
Change of 2.5%	–	70[e]
Change of 5%	–	140
Change of 10%	–	280

Sources: a = Summary estimate from time-series data (Loomis, 1999; Gouveia, 2000; Conceiao, 2000; Saldiva, 1994; Ostro, 1999)
b = Saldiva et al, 1995; Ostro et al, 1996; Borja-Aburto et al, 1997; Tellez-Rojo et al, 1997, 2000; Hong et al, 1999
c = Tellez-Rojo et al, 1997
d = Ilabaca et al, 1999
e = Romieu et al, 1996

al, 1998; Ilabaca et al, 1999; Gouveia et al, 2000; Romero et al, 2001) (Table 3.1). The fact that exposed children in developing countries often suffer from additional risk factors such as poor living conditions and nutrition deficiency increases their susceptibility to the adverse effects of particulate pollution.

Chronic exposure

Chronic cough, bronchitis and chest illness (but not asthma) have been associated with various measures of particulate air pollution. Results suggest that a $10\mu g/m^3$ increase in PM_{10} is associated with a 5 to 25 per cent increase in bronchitis or chronic cough, in adults as well as children (Pope and Dockery, 1999). The impact of chronic particulate exposure has also been observed on lung functions. The results suggest that a $10\mu g/m^3$ increase in PM_{10} was associated with only a small decline (1 to 3 per cent) in lung function (Pope and Dockery, 1999). Recent results suggest that exposure to air pollution may lead to a reduction in maximum attained lung function, which occurs early in adult life, and ultimately to an increased risk of chronic respiratory illness during adulthood (Berkey et al, 1986; Gaudermann et al, 2000).

Some recent studies have focused on the impact of air pollution on fetal growth, pre-term birth, birth weight and other pregnancy outcomes because of the increasing concern that air pollution might affect fetal development. Significant exposure–response relationships between maternal exposure to SO_2 and to total suspended particulates (TSP) and low birth weight were observed in studies conducted in China (Wang et al, 1997) and the Czech Republic (Boback et al, 2000); relationships also exist between these pollutants and fetal growth retardation (Delmeek et al, 1999) and pre-term birth (Ritz et al, 2000). These findings may indicate harmful effects of lasting significance because low birth weight and fetal growth retardation have been linked to altered respiratory health later in life (Gold et al, 1999), and fetal growth retardation may lead to an increased susceptibility to air pollution exposure and other environmental factors (Ashworth et al, 1998).

HEALTH EFFECTS OF OZONE

Ozone is a colourless reactive oxidant that occurs with other photochemical oxidants and fine particles in the complex mixture commonly called 'smog', as discussed in Chapter 2. Ozone is a strong oxidant, formed in ground level ambient air by a complex series of reactions involving volatile organic compounds, sunlight and nitrogen oxides (WHO, 2000).

The toxicology of ozone has been investigated extensively, as discussed in Chapter 2. The main health concern of exposure to ozone is its effect on the respiratory system; most of the studies on the health effects of ozone have focused on short term exposures (Table 3.2).

Mortality

Results of time-series studies on associations between ozone and daily mortality have been inconsistent (Loomis et al, 1996; Hong et al, 1999; Tellez-Rojo et al, 2000). However, recent studies have reported a significant association between ozone and daily mortality counts during the high ozone season (Thurston and Ito, 1999; Samet et al, 2000; Hoek et al, 2000; Cifuentes et al, 2000).

Table 3.2 *Health outcomes associated with changes in peak daily ambient ozone concentration in epidemiological studies*

Health effect indicators	Changes in 1-h O_3 ($\mu g/m^3$)[a]
Daily morbidity (upper respiratory illnesses)	
Change of 5%	25[b]
Change of 10%	50
Change of 20%	100
Daily morbidity (emergency visits for asthma among children)	
Change of 5%	20[c]
Change of 10%	40
Change of 20%	80
Exacerbation of respiratory symptoms in children with moderate asthma	
Change of 5%	30[d]
Change of 10%	60
Change of 20%	120
Peak expiratory flow rate in children with moderate asthma	
Change of 2.5%	185[d]
Change of 5%	370

Note: 1-h = hourly average.
Sources: a = 1$\mu g/m^3$ = 0.5ppb
b = Tellez-Rojo et al, 1997
c = Castillejos et al, 1995
d = Romieu et al, 1996; Romieu et al, 1997

Morbidity

Epidemiological studies have documented a number of acute effects including increases in emergency visits and hospital admissions due to respiratory diseases, increase in respiratory symptoms (such as cough, throat dryness, eye and chest discomfort, thoracic pain and headache) and temporary lung function decrements (Lippmann, 1989; American Thoracic Society, 1996; Nyberg and Pershagen, 1996; Thurston and Ito, 1999). Ozone exposure is a risk factor for the exacerbation of symptoms in asthmatic subjects (Romieu, 1996, 1997; Thurston and Ito, 1999). More importantly, a recent study has linked ozone exposure to the incidence of new diagnosis asthma in children having heavy exercise activities in communities with high ozone concentration (McConnell et al, 2002).

Studies conducted in Mexico City, where ozone levels frequently exceed by a large margin the WHO guidelines, have documented an increase in asthma-related emergency visits, a decrease in peak expiratory flow rate and an increase in respiratory symptoms in asthmatic children (Romieu et al, 1997). In addition, studies conducted in Mexico and Southern California have reported an association between ozone exposure and school absenteeism for respiratory illnesses, even at levels of exposure that are common in many urban areas (average 20 to 50ppb, 10am to 6pm) (Romieu et al, 1997; Gilliland et al, 2001).

Because ozone is a potent oxidant, anti-oxidant supplementation could modulate the impact of ozone exposure on the respiratory tract. Results from recent studies suggest that increasing the dietary intake of anti-oxidant vitamins (beta-carotene, vitamin E and vitamin C) may protect against the acute adverse effects of ozone exposure (Romieu et al, 1998, 2000). This finding is important because micronutrient deficiency is prevalent in many developing countries and may enhance the adverse effect of air pollutant exposure, in particular, in populations that are chronically exposed.

As for many other pollutants, there is major concern in relation to the long term effects of ozone. Many children in developing nations are exposed to high levels of ozone on a daily basis. The health implications of this exposure are still unclear, but there is good reason for concern: ozone exposure induces inflammatory responses and long term exposure to high levels of ozone could lead to chronic impairment of lung function (Lippmann, 1993).

HEALTH EFFECTS OF NITROGEN DIOXIDE

The major sources of anthropogenic emissions of nitrogen dioxide (NO_2) into the atmosphere are motor vehicles and stationary sources, such as electric utility plants and industrial boilers. NO_2 is highly reactive and has been reported to cause bronchitis and pneumonia, as well as to increase susceptibility to respiratory infections (Table 3.3). NO_2 has been shown to affect both the cellular and humoral immune system, and to impair immune responses. A review of epidemiological studies suggests that children exposed to NO_2 are at increased risk of respiratory illness (Hasselblad et al, 1992). NO_2 has also been associated with daily mortality in children less than five years old (Saldiva, 1994) and intra-uterine mortality levels in Sao Paulo, Brazil (Pereira, 1998). In these reports, NO_2 was more significantly associated than the other pollutants that were studied. Recently, longitudinal data from the Children's Health Study, conducted in 12 communities of Southern California, suggest a significant deficit in lung growth related to NO_2 and fine particulate exposure (Gaudermann, 2000).

The interdependence between NO_2 and other pollutants observed in various studies suggests that the observed health effects could be related to the interplay among contaminants from combustion sources.

HEALTH EFFECTS OF CARBON MONOXIDE

Carbon monoxide (CO) is one of the most common and widely distributed air pollutants. It is a product of the incomplete combustion of carbon-containing materials, in particular fossil fuel. Carbon monoxide enters the bloodstream and reduces the delivery of oxygen to the body's organs and tissues. People who suffer from cardiovascular disease, particularly those with angina or peripheral vascular disease, are much more susceptible to the health effects of CO.

Table 3.3 *Health outcome associated with NO_2 exposure in epidemiological studies*

Health effect	Mechanism
Increased incidence of respiratory infections	Reduced efficacy of lung defences
Increased severity of respiratory infections	Reduced efficacy of lung defences
Respiratory symptoms	Airways injury
Reduced lung function	Airways and alveolar injury
Worsening clinical status of persons with asthma, chronic obstructive pulmonary disease or other chronic respiratory conditions	Airways injury

Source: Romieu, 1999

Carbon monoxide leads to a decreased oxygen uptake capacity with decreased work capacity under maximum exercise conditions. Inhalation of CO leads to an increased concentration of carboxyhaemoglobin in the blood. According to available data (Table 3.4), the concentration of carboxyhaemoglobin in the blood required to induce a decreased oxygen uptake capacity is approximately 5 per cent. An impairment in the ability to judge correctly slight differences in successive short time intervals has been observed at lower carboxyhaemoglobin levels of 3.2 to 4.2 per cent. The classic symptoms of CO poisoning are headache and dizziness at carboxyhaemoglobin levels between 10 and 30 per cent. At carboxyhaemoglobin levels higher than about 30 per cent, the symptoms are severe headaches, cardiovascular symptoms and malaise. Above carboxyhaemoglobin levels of roughly 40 per cent, there is considerable risk of coma and death (Romieu, 1999).

Epidemiological studies relating CO with daily counts of mortality or hospital admissions need to be interpreted with caution. In contrast with other pollutants, CO measurements from fixed monitors (used for air surveillance) correlate poorly with CO levels measured at the personal level. However, various studies in developed countries have documented significant association between daily variations in CO and an increase in premature mortality or hospitalizations from congestive heart failure (Schwartz, 1995; Burnett et al, 1998). Few studies have been reported from developing countries. However, limited data from Sao Paulo, Brazil suggest that CO exposure is prevalent and may be associated with intra-uterine death (Pereira et al, 1998) and with pre-term birth (Ritz et al, 2000).

HEALTH EFFECTS OF LEAD

Lead poisoning is one of the most important problems of environmental and occupational origin, because of its high prevalence and persistence of toxicity in affected populations. Lead poisoning may alter virtually all biochemical processes and organ systems in humans. Lead can interfere with the cardiovascular and reproductive systems, with the blood formation process, with vitamin D function and with neurological processes, among others (Howson et al, 1995). Of special concern has been the accumulation of

Table 3.4 *Health effects associated with low-level carbon monoxide exposure, based on carboxyhaemoglobin levels*

Carboxyhaemoglobin concentration (%)	Effects
2.3–4.3	Decrease (3–7%) in the relation between work time and exhaustion in exercising young healthy adults
2.0–4.5	Decrease in exercise capacity in patients with angina (cardiovascular impairment)
5–5.5	Decrease in maximum oxygen consumption and exercise in young healthy men during strenuous exercise
<5	Vigilance decrement
5–17	Decrease of visual perception, manual dexterity, ability to learn or performance in complex sensorimotor tasks (eg driving)

Source: Romieu, 1999

experimental and epidemiological evidence suggesting that lead is a neurotoxin that impairs brain development in children, even at levels that were previously considered safe (Needleman and Bellinger, 1991). Studies conducted in Mexico and China have documented similar effects (Munoz et al, 1993; Shen et al, 1996).

The toxic effects associated with chronic low level lead exposure are a major concern, especially as there are no clinical symptoms that will allow the prompt recognition of lead intoxication; yet lead exposure is preventable through the identification and control of sources of exposure. Beginning in the 1970s, many countries initiated regulatory and legislative efforts to prevent lead exposure. Regulatory actions have been targeted to reduce the use of leaded paints, to eliminate lead from gasoline and to control large industrial point source emissions. These interventions have resulted in important reductions in lead exposure. For example, in Mexico City the introduction of unleaded gasoline in 1990 was associated with a decline in lead ambient concentrations from an annual average of $1.2\mu g/m^3$ to an annual average of $0.2\mu g/m^3$ in 1993 (Hernandez-Avila, 1997), as well as with an estimated decline of 7.6 micrograms per decilitre ($\mu g/dl$) in the mean blood lead of children (Rothenberg et al, 1998). In South Africa from 1984 to 1990 (Maresky and Grobler, 1993) a reduction of the lead content in gasoline was also reported to be associated with a significant decrease in blood lead levels from 9.7 micrograms per decilitre ($\mu g/dl$) to $7.2\mu g/dl$.

Although lead exposure is recognized as an important public health problem, there are few studies published from developing countries (Table 3.5). Furthermore, most published studies have not evaluated exposure among children aged 24 months to 6 years, who are at higher risk of exposure and of suffering the health effects of lead exposure. Therefore, the real magnitude of the problem remains unknown.

Control of lead exposure in developing countries will require additional efforts and properly targeted interventions to account for the particular condition in which exposure takes place.

Table 3.5 *Recent published studies describing blood lead levels in developing countries*

Author, journal and year of publication	City and country	Age group (years)	Population studied	Sample size	Sources of exposure identified	Blood levels in µg/dl
Song, H Q (1993)	Beijing, China	5–6	Children	128	Air & food	7.7
Hwang, Y H (1990)	Taipei, China	At birth	Newborns	205	Air lead	7.4
Saxena, D K (1994)	Lucknow, India	At birth	Newborns		Not identified	16.9
Vijayalakshmi, P (1996)	Chennai, India	26–55	Office workers	10		4.1
			Autoshop workers	9	Gasoline & ambient air	17.5
			Bus drivers	22		12.1
			Traffic police	88		11.2
Counter, S A (1997)	Rural communities, Ecuador	4–15	Children	82	Battery recycling	52.6
Schutz, A (1997)	Montevideo, Uruguay	2–14	Children	96	Exposure to traffic	9.5
Lopez, L (1996)	Mexico City, Mexico	1–5	Children	603	Ambient air, lead glazed ceramics	15.0
Romieu, I (1995)		1–5	Children	200	Ambient air, lead glazed ceramics	9.9
Gonzalez, T (1997)		At birth	Children	238	Ambient air, lead glazed ceramics	7.1
Farias, P (1996)		13–43	Pregnant women	513	Ambient air, lead glazed ceramics	11.08
Ramirez, A V (1997)	Lima, Peru Huancayo, Peru La Oroya, Peru Yaupi, Peru	18–50	Adult	320	Degree of industrialization	26.9 22.4 34.8 14.0
Niagu, J (1997)	Durban, Metropolitan region Vulamehlo, South Africa	3–10	Children	1200	Ambient air	10.0 3.8

CONCLUSIONS

Epidemiological data collected in developed countries suggest that air pollution affects both mortality and morbidity rates, and generates high social costs associated with premature death and a decrease in the quality of life. In these countries, large quantities of resources are targeted for clean-ups and remedial actions, and safety standards and regulations are becoming stricter. In contrast, developing countries are trapped in the trade-offs of economic growth and environmental protection. Air pollution occurs jointly with other important public health problems, a situation that inhibits the adequate targeting of resources for remediation or prevention of environmental problems. Furthermore, policy-makers may favour employment or economic growth over environment.

Direct extrapolation of health effects observed in populations living in urban areas of developed countries to populations living in urban areas of developing countries is difficult. For example, it is likely that the neurotoxic effect of lead will be similar for Mexican or Australian children living in similar conditions. However, the concurrent existence of iron deficiency and lead exposure in Mexican children could increase the toxicity of lead. Similarly, other variables such as population structure, as well as exposure to other pollutants, may preclude direct extrapolation (Romieu and Borja-Aburto, 1997). Nonetheless, most available evidence suggests that populations living in cities with high levels of air pollution in developing countries experience similar or greater adverse effects of air pollution. Certainly, more information is needed to assess the health effects of air pollution in these countries and efforts should be targeted to increase the number of epidemiological studies.

The World Health Organization has established guidelines (WHO, 2000) for ambient air pollution levels that set the acceptable levels of the risk of adverse effects. The use of these criteria may serve as a long term objective for countries initiating air pollution control programmes and as a base for the development of national standards and regulations.

Vehicular exhaust is considered in great part responsible for the health effects related to air pollutants. Although current fossil fuel use in developing countries is still half that of developed countries, it is expected to increase by 120 per cent by the year 2010. Several estimates have been conducted at the national and international levels to determine the impact of control programmes on health benefits. Recently, Kuenzli et al (2000) estimated that in three European countries, air pollution caused 6 per cent of total mortality or 40,000 attributable cases per year. About half of all mortality caused by air pollution was attributed to motorized traffic (Kuenzli et al, 2000). Another estimate assessing the health benefits of urban air pollution reduction associated with climate change mitigation in four cities (Santiago, Sao Paulo, Mexico City and New York City) reported that the adoption of readily available technologies to lessen fossil fuel emissions over the next two decades in these four cities would reduce particulate and ozone, as well as avoid approximately 64,000 premature deaths, 65,000 cases of chronic bronchitis and 37 million person-days of work lost or other restricted activity (Cifuentes et al, 2001). In agreement with these results, a recent estimate for Delhi, India suggests that an annual reduction of $100\mu g/m^3$ in TSP could be associated with a reduction of about 1400 premature deaths per year (Cropper et al, 1997).

There is an urgent need for the implementation of control programmes to reduce levels of particulate and other pollutant emissions. To be effective, these programmes should include the participation of the different stakeholders and initiate activities to identify and characterize air pollution problems, as well as to estimate potential health impacts. A full understanding of the problem and its potential consequences for the local setting is essential for effectively targeting interventions to reduce the harmful impacts of air pollution in human populations.

REFERENCES

American Thoracic Society (ATS) (1996) 'A committee of the environmental and occupational health assembly of the American Thoracic Society. State of the art review: health effects of outdoor air pollution' in *American Review of Critical Care Medicine*, vol 153, no 1, pp33–50, and vol 153, no 2, pp477–998

Ashworth, A (1998) 'Effects of intrauterine growth retardation on mortality and morbidity in infants and young children' in *European Journal of Clinical Nutrition*, vol 52, ppS34–41

Berkey, C, Ware, J, Dockery, D, Ferris, B J and Speizer, F (1986) 'Indoor air pollution and pulmonary function growth in preadolescent children' in *American Journal of Epidemiology*, vol 123, pp250–260

Bobak, M (2000) 'Outdoor air pollution, low birth weight, and prematurity' in *Environmental Health Perspective*, vol 108, no 2, pp173–176

Borja-Aburto, V H, Loomis, D P, Barígdiwala, S I, Shy, C M and Rascón Pacheco, R A (1997) 'Ozone, suspended particulates and daily mortality in Mexico City' in *American Journal of Epidemiology*, vol 145, pp258–268

Burnett, R T, Cakmak, S and Brook, J R (1998) 'The effect of the urban ambient air pollution mix on daily mortality rates in 11 Canadian cities' in *Canadian Journal of Public Health (Revue Canadienne de Santé Publique)*, vol 89, pp152–156

Burnett, R T, Cakmak, S, Raizenne, M E, Stieb, D, Vincent, R, Krewski, D, Brook, J R, Philips, O and Ozkaynak, (1998) 'The association between ambient carbon monoxide levels and daily mortality in Toronto, Canada' in *Journal of the Air and Waste Management Association*, vol 48, pp689–700

Castillejos, M, Gold, D R, Damokosh, A I, Serrano, P, Allen, G, McDonnell, W F, Dockery, D, Ruiz, Velasco S, Hernandez-Avila, M and Hayes, C (1995) 'Acute effects of ozone on the pulmonary function of exercising schoolchildren from Mexico City' in *American Journal of Respiratory and Critical Care Medicine,* vol 152, pp1501–1507

Cifuentes, L A, Vega, J, Kopfer, K and Lave, L B (2000) 'Effect of the fine fraction of particulate matter versus the coarse mass and other pollutants on daily mortality in Santiago, Chile' in *Journal of Air & Waste Management Association*, vol 50, pp1287–1298

Cifuentes, L, Borja-Aburto, V H, Gouveia, N, Thurston, G and Davis, D L (2001) 'Assessing the health benefits of urban air pollution reduction associated with climate change mitigation (2000–2020): Santiago, Sao Paulo, Mexico City, and New York City' in *Environmental Health Perspectives*, vol 109, suppl 3, pp419–425

Cohen, A J and Nikula, K (1999) 'The health effects of diesel exhaust' in S T Holgate et al (eds) *Air Pollution and Health*, Academic Press, London, pp707–745

Conceiao, G M S, Miraglia, S G E K, Kishi, H S, Saldiva, P N H and Singer, J M (2001) 'Air pollution and child mortality: a time series study in Sao Paulo, Brazil' in *Environmental Health Perspectives*, vol 109, no 3, pp347–350

Cropper, M L, Simon, N B, Alberini, A and Sharma, P K (1997) *The Health Effects of Air Pollution in Delhi, India,* PRI Working Paper 1860, World Bank, Washington, DC

Delmeek, J, Selevan, S G, Benes, I, Solansky, I and Sram, R J (1999) 'Fetal growth and maternal exposure to particulate matter during pregnancy' in *Environmental Health Perspectives*, vol 107, no 6, pp475–480

Diaz-Sanchez, D, Garcia, M P, Wang, M, Jyrala, M and Saxon, A (1999) 'Nasal challenge with diesel exhaust particles can induce sensitization to a neoallergen in the human mucosa' in *Journal of Allergy & Clinical Immunology*, vol 104, no 6, pp1183–1188

Dockery, D W, Pope, A, Xu, X, Spengler, J D, Ware, J H, Fay, M E, Ferris, B G and Speizer, F E (1993) 'An association between air pollution and mortality in six US cities' in *New England Journal of Medicine*, vol 329, no 24, pp173-179

EPA (1996) 'National ambient air quality standards for particulate matter: proposed rule' in *Federal Register,* vol 61, no 241, 40CFR part 50

Gauderman, W J, McConnell, R, Gilliland, F, London, S, Thomas, D, Avol, E, Vora, H, Berhane, K, Rappaport, E B, Lurmann, F, Margolis, H G and Peters, J (2000) 'Association between air pollution and lung function growth in southern California children' in *American Journal of Respiratory and Critical Care Medicine*, vol 162, pp1383–1399

Gilliland, F D, Berhane, K, Rappaport, E B, Thomas, D C, Avol, E, Gauderman, W J, London, S J, Margolis, H G, McConnell, R, Islam, K T and Peters, J M (2001) 'The effects of ambient air pollution on school absenteeism due to respiratory illnesses' in *Epidemiology,* vol 12, no 1, pp43–54

Gold, D R, Burge, H A, Carey, V, Milton, D K, Platts-Mills, T and Weiss, S T (1999) 'Predictors of repeated wheeze in the first year of life: the relative roles of cockroaches, birth weight, acute lower respiratory illness, and maternal smoking' in *American Journal of Respiratory and Critical Care Medicine,* vol 160, pp227–236

Gouveia, N and Fletcher, T (2000) 'Time series analysis of air pollution and mortality: effects by cause, age and socioeconomic status' in *Journal of Epidemiology Community Health,* vol 54, pp750–755

Hasselblad, V, Eddy, D M and Kotchmar, D J (1992) 'Synthesis of environmental evidence: nitrogen dioxide epidemiological studies' in *Journal of Air Waste Management Association*, vol 5, pp662–671

Health Effect Institute (HEI) (1988) *Air Pollution, the Automobile and Public Health*, Health Effects Institute, National Academic Press, Washington, DC

Hernandez-Avila, M (1997) 'El plomo: un problema en la salud pública en México. Intoxicación por plomo en México: Prevención y Control' in M Hernandez-Avila and E Palazuelos Rendon (eds) *Perspectivas en Salud Pública,* pp13–24

Hoek, G, Schwartz, J D, Groot, B and Eilers, P (1997) 'Effects of ambient particulate matter and ozone on daily mortality in Rotterdam, The Netherlands' in *Archives of Environmental Health*, vol 52, no 6, pp455–463

Holdren, J P and Smith, K R (2000) 'Energy, the environment and health' in Goldemburg (ed) *World Energy Assessment: Energy and the Challenge of Sustainability*, UNDP, New York, pp61–110

Hong, Y C, Leem, J H, Ha, E H and Christiani, D C (1999) 'PM[10] exposure, gaseous pollutants, and daily mortality in Inchon, South Korea' in *Environmental Health Perspectives*, vol 107, pp873–878

Howson, P C, Hernandez-Avila, M and Rall, D A (eds) (1995) *Lead in the Americas – A Call for Action,* Institute of Medicine, National Academy of Sciences and National Institute of Public Health (Mexico)

Ilabaca, M, Olaeta, I, Campos, E, Villaire, J, Téllez-Rojo, M M and Romieu, I (1999) 'Association between levels of fine particulate and emergency visits for pneumonia and other respiratory illnesses among children in Santiago, Chile' in *Journal of Air Waste Management Association,* vol 48, pp174–183

Klemm, R J, Mason, R M, Heilig, C M, Neas, L M and Dockery, D (2000) 'Is daily mortality associated specifically with fine particles? Data reconstruction and replication of analyses' in *Journal of Air Waste Management Association,* vol 50, pp1215–1222

Kuenzli, N, Kaiser, R, Medina, S, Studnicka, M, Chamel, O, Filliger, P, Herry, M, Horak, F, Puybonnieux-Texier, V, Quenel, P, Schneider, J, Seethaler, R, Vergnaud, J C and Sommer, H (2000) 'Public health impact of outdoors and traffic-related air pollution: a European assessment' in *Lancet,* vol 356, pp795–801

Krzyzanowski, M and Schwela, D (1999) 'Patterns of air pollution in developing countries' in S T Holgate et al (eds), *Air Pollution and Health,* Academic Press, London, pp105–113

Lacasaña, M, Romieu, I and Aguilar, C (1999) 'Evolución de la contaminación del aire e impacto de los programas de control en tres megaciudades de América Latina' in *Salud Pública de México,* vol 41, pp203–215

Lippmann, M (1989) 'Effects of ozone on respiratory function and structure' in *Annual Review of Public Health,* vol 10, pp49–67

Lippmann, M (1993) 'Health effects of tropospheric ozone: a review of recent research findings and their implications to ambient air quality standards' in *Journal of Exposure Analysis and Environmental Epidemiology,* vol 3, pp103–129

Loomis, D, Castillejos, M, Gold, D R et al (1999) 'Air pollution and infant mortality in Mexico City' in *Epidemiology,* vol 10, pp118–123

Loomis, D P, Borja-Aburto, V H, Barígdiwala, S I and Shy, C M (1996) 'Ozone exposure and daily mortality in Mexico City: a time-series analysis, research report' in *Health Effects Institute,* vol 75, pp1–37, discussion pp39–45

Maresky, L S and Grobler, S R (1993) 'Effect of the reduction of petrol lead on the blood lead levels of South Africans' in *Science of the Total Environment,* vol 136, pp43–48

McConnell, R, Berhane, K, Gilliland, F, London, S, Islam, T, Gauderman, W J, Avol, E, Margolis, H G and Peters, J M 'Asthma in exercising children exposed to ozone: a cohort study' in *The Lancet,* vol 359, pp386–391

Munoz, H, Romieu, L, Palazuelos, E, Mancillasanchez, T, Menesesgonzalez, F and Hernandez-Avila, M (1993) 'Blood lead level and neurobehavioral development among children living in Mexico City' in *Archives of Environmental Health,* vol 48, pp132–139

Needleman, H L and Bellinger, D (1991) 'The health effects of low level exposure to lead' in *Annual Review of Public Health,* vol 12, pp111–140

Nyberg, F and Pershagen, G (1996) 'Epidemiologic studies on ozone' in *Scandinavian Journal of Work, Environment and Health,* vol 22 (suppl), pp72–98

Ostro, B, Chestnut, L, Vichit-Vadakan, and Laixuthai, A (1999) 'The impact of fine particulate matter on daily mortality in Bangkok, Thailand' in J Chow et al (eds) *PM[2.5]: A Fine Particulate Standard,* vol II, Long Beach, CA, pp939–949

Ostro, B, Sanchez, J M, Aranda, C and Eskeland, G (1996) 'Air pollution and mortality: results from a study of Santiago, Chile' in *Journal of Exposure Environmental Epidemiology,* vol 6, no 1, pp97–114

Pereira, L A, Loomis, D, Conceicao, G M, Braga, A L F, Arcas, R M, Kishi, H S, Singer, J M, Bohm, G M and Saldiva, P H (1998) 'Association between air pollution and intrauterine mortality in Sao Paulo, Brazil' in *Environmental Health Perspectives*, vol 106, pp325–329

Pino, P, Romieu, I, Villegas, R, Walter, T and Oyarzún, M (1998) 'Wheezing bronchitis in infants: influence of airborne fine particulate matter and environmental tabacco smoke exposure' in *American Journal of Respiratory Critical Care and Medicine*, A877

Pope III, C A and Dockery, D (1999) 'Epidemiology of particle effects' in S T Holgate et al (eds) *Air Pollution and Health*, Academic Press, London, pp671–705

Pope III, C A (2000) 'Epidemiology of fine particulate air pollution and human health: biologic mechanisms and who's at risk?' in *Environmental Health Perspectives*, vol 108, no 4, pp713–723

Pope III, C A, Thun, M J, Namboodiri, M M, Dockery, D W, Evans, J S, Speizer, F E and Heath, C W Jr (1995) 'Particulate air pollution as a predictor of mortality in a prospective study of US adults' in *American Journal of Respiratory and Critical Care Medicine*, vol 151, pp669–674

Ritz, B, Yu, F, Chapa, G and Fruin, S (2000) 'Effect of air pollution on preterm birth among children in southern California between 1989 and 1993' in *Epidemiology*, vol 11, no 5, pp502–511

Romero-Placeres, M, Mas-Bermejo, P, Lacasaña-Navarro, M, Tellez-Rojo, M M, Aguilar-Valdes, J and Romieu, I (in press) 'Contaminación atmosférica, crisis aguda de asma bronquial e infecciones respiratorias agudas en menores cubanos', *Salud Pública de México*

Romieu, I, Lugo, M C, Velasco, S R, Sanchez, S, Meneses, F and Hernandez-Avila, M (1992) 'Air pollution and school absenteeism among children in Mexico City' in *American Journal of Epidemiology*, vol 136, no 12, pp1524–1531

Romieu, I (1999) 'Epidemiological studies of health effects arising from motor vehicle air pollution' in D Schwella and O Zali (eds) *Urban Traffic Pollution*, Ecotox/WHO/E & F N Spon, London and New York, pp9–49

Romieu, I and Borja-Aburto, V (1997) 'Particulate air pollution and daily mortality: can results be generalized to Latin American countries?' in *Salud Pública de México*, vol 39, pp403–411

Romieu, I, Meneses, F, Ramirez, M, Ruiz, S, Perez Padilla, R, Sienra, J J, Gerber, M, Grievink, L, Dekker, R, Walda, I and Brunekreff, B (1998) 'Antioxidant supplementation and respiratory functions among workers exposed to high levels of ozone' in *American Journal of Respiratory Critical and Care Medicine*, vol 158, pp226–232

Romieu, I, Meneses, F, Ruiz, S, Huerta, J, Sienra, J J, White, M, Etzel, R and Hernandez-Avila, M (1997) 'Effects of intermittent ozone exposure on peak expiratory flow and respiratory symptoms among asthmatic children in Mexico City' in *Archives of Environmental Health*, vol 52, no 5, pp368–376

Romieu, I, Meneses, F, Ruiz, S, Sienra, J J, Huerta, J, White, M and Etzel, R (1996) 'Effects of air pollution on the respiratory health of asthmatic children living in Mexico City' in *American Journal of Respiratory and Critical Care Medicine*, vol 154, pp300–307

Romieu, I, Weizenfeld, H and Finkleman, J (1990) 'Urban air pollution in Latin America and the Caribbean: health perspectives' in *World Health Statistics Quarterly*, vol 43, pp154–268

Rothenberg, S L, Schnaas, L, Perroni, E, Hernandez, R M and Karchmer, S (1998) 'Secular trends in blood lead levels in a cohort of Mexico City children' in *Archives of Environmental Health*, vol 53, pp231–235

Saldiva, P H N, Lichtenfels, A J F C, Paiva, P S O et al (1994) 'Association between air pollution and mortality due to respiratory diseases in children in Sao Paulo, Brazil: a preliminary report' in *Environ Research,* vol 65, pp218–225

Saldiva, P H N, Pope, C A III, Schwartz, J, Dockery, D W, Lichtenfelds, A J, Salge, J M, Barone, Y and Bohm, G M (1995) 'Air pollution and mortality in elderly people: a time series study in Sao Paulo, Brazil' in *Archives of Environmental Health*, vol 50, pp159–163

Samet, J M, Dominici, F, Curreiro, F C, Coursac, I and Zeger, S L (2000) 'Fine particulate air pollution and mortality in 20 US cities, 1987–1994' in *New England Journal of Medicine*, vol 343, pp1742–1749

Schwartz, J, Dockery, D W and Neas, L M (1996) 'Is daily mortality associated specifically with fine particulates?' in *Journal of Air & Waste Management Association*, vol 46, pp927–939

Schwartz, J and Zanobetti, A (2000) 'Using meta-smoothing to estimate dose–response trends across multiple studies with application to air pollution and daily death' in *Epidemiology*, vol 11, pp666–672

Schwartz, J (1995) 'Is carbon monoxide a risk factor for hospital admission for heart failure?' in *American Journal of Public Health*, vol 85, no 10, pp1343–1345

Shen, X, Yan, C and Zhou, J (1996) 'Relationship between lead content in umbilical blood and neurobehavioral development in infants' in *Chinese Journal of Preventive Medicine* (in Chinese), vol 30, pp68–70

Tellez-Rojo, M M, Romieu, I, Ruiz-Velasco, S, Lezana, M A and Hernandez-Avila, M M (2000) 'Daily respiratory mortality and PM[10] pollution in Mexico City: importance of considering place of death' in *European Respiratory Journal*, vol 16, pp391–396

Tellez-Rojo, M M, Romieu, I, Pena, M P, Ruiz-Velasco, S, Meneses-Gonzales, F and Hernandez-Avila, M (1997) 'Efecto de la contaminación ambiental sobre las consultas por infecciones respiratorias en niños de la Ciudad de México' in *Salud Pública de México,* vol 39, no 6, pp513–522

Thomas, P T and Zelikoff, J T (1999) 'Air pollutants: modulators of pulmonary host resistance against infection' in S T Holgate et al (eds) *Air Pollution and Health*, Academic Press, London, pp357–379

Thurston, G D and Ito, K (1999) 'Epidemiological studies of ozone exposure effects' in S T Holgate et al (eds) *Air Pollution and Health*, Academic Press, London, pp485–510

Wang, X, Ding, H, Ryan, L and Xu, X (1997) 'Association between air pollution and low birth weight: a community-based study' in *Environmental Health Perspective*, vol 105, no 5, pp514–520

WHO (World Health Organization) (1993) *The Urban Health Crisis: Strategies for Health for All in the Face of Rapid Urbanization,* Report of WHO Expert Committee, WHO, Geneva

WHO (World Health Organization) (1997) *Healthy Cities Air Management,* WHO, Geneva

WHO (World Health Organization) (2000) *Air Quality Guidelines for Europe,* WHO Regional Office for Europe, Copenhagen

Woodruff, T, Grillo, J and Schoendorf, K G (1997) 'The relationship between selected causes of postneonatal infant mortality and particulate air pollution in the United States' in *Environmental Health Perspective*, vol 105, no 6, pp608–612

Zeger, S L, Dominici, F and Samet, J (1999) 'Harvesting-resistant estimates of air pollution effects on mortality' in *Epidemiology*, vol 10, pp171–175

4

Local Ambient Air Quality Management

Dietrich Schwela

ABSTRACT

The aim of local ambient air quality management is to protect public health and the environment from the damaging effects of air pollution, and to eliminate or reduce to a minimum human exposure to hazardous pollutants. In developed countries air quality management has used sophisticated instruments to determine the necessary measures to control polluting sources. This has taken the form of clean air implementation plans based on an evaluation of the most efficient method to reduce air pollution. In contrast, an assessment of the air pollutant reduction measures in developing countries is typically based on more limited information concerning local sources, the dispersion of air pollution, actual air pollutant levels and related adverse effects. The lack of emissions inventories and air quality standards makes assessment difficult. The World Health Organization (WHO) has produced guidelines for air quality to assist developing countries to determine the best measures to abate air pollution with limited information. This has been achieved by drawing upon knowledge gained in developed countries and giving practical advice on how to develop legally enforceable air quality standards and simplified clean air implementation plans. The guidelines provide advice on which legal aspects need to be considered, how adverse effects in the population at risk can be defined, how exposure–response relationships can be applied and how acceptable levels of risks can be assessed. The air quality guidelines provide advice on the health effects of air pollution under different geographical, social, economic and cultural conditions and how the capability for implementing air quality standards may be increased. The Air Management Information System (AMIS), set up by WHO in 1997, is an additional information source on air pollution concentrations in major and megacities, air quality standards in various countries, air quality management capabilities and the instruments used in various cities of developed and developing countries. This chapter discusses the factors that need to be considered in local air quality management and the guidance provided by the WHO guidelines for air quality and AMIS. Recent developments in international programmes on air quality such as the EU CAFE programme are also considered.

INTRODUCTION

This chapter discusses the various aspects of local air quality management in developing countries, including the conversion of WHO air quality guidelines to national air quality standards, their use in local air quality management, and the assistance that AMIS can provide (WHO, 1997a, 1998a, 2001). The WHO air quality guidelines for Europe (WHO/EURO, 1987) have been of major support to countries undertaking risk assessment and setting national standards. The guidelines have been updated, revised (WHO/EURO, 2000) and made globally applicable by taking into account factors that might be influential to the health outcome in other regions (WHO, 2000; Schwela, 2000a, 2000b). The application of the guidelines for the setting of national air quality standards has been extensively discussed in two publications (de Koning, 1987; WHO, 1998b; see also WHO, 2000).

In order to understand the difference between air quality guidelines and air quality standards, these terms are defined as follows:

An *air quality guideline* is any kind of recommendation or guidance on the protection of a population of human beings or receptors in the environment (eg vegetation, materials) from the adverse effects of air pollutants. Air quality guidelines are exclusively based on exposure–response relationships found in epidemiological, toxicological and environment-related studies. An air quality guideline is not restricted to a numerical value, and may express exposure–response information or unit risks in different ways.

An *air quality guideline value* is a fixed numerical value corresponding to a defined averaging time. It is expressed as a concentration in ambient air, a deposition level or some other physico-chemical value. In the case of human health, the air quality guideline is a concentration below which no adverse effects are expected, although a small residual risk always exists. Compliance of appropriate statistical location parameters with a guideline value does not guarantee that effects do not occur.

An *air quality standard* is a level of air pollutant (concentration, deposition etc) that is promulgated by a regulatory authority and adopted as legally enforceable. In addition to the effect-based level and the averaging time of a guideline value, several elements have to be specified in the formulation of a standard. These include the measurement procedure, definition of compliance parameters corresponding to the averaging times and the permitted number of exceedances.

The WHO air quality guidelines provide a basis for protecting public health from the adverse effects of environmental pollutants, and for eliminating or reducing to a minimum contaminants that are known or likely to be hazardous to human health and wellbeing (WHO/EURO, 1987). Air quality guidelines provide background information and guidance to governments in making risk management decisions, particularly in setting standards. They also assist governments to undertake local control measures in the framework of air quality management.

The updated and revised, globally applicable air quality guidelines of WHO are presented in Tables 4.1, 4.2 and 4.3. These guideline values do not include guideline values for suspended particulate matter. In deriving the air quality guidelines it was argued that a threshold for this compound including the size-dependent fractions PM_{10} and $PM_{2.5}$ could not be established and consequently no guideline value be given. Instead it is recommended to use Figures 4.1, 4.2 and 4.3 for fixing an acceptable risk for some health endpoint in the sense of a risk consideration. The percentage change in some health endpoint indicated in these figures is related to the risk of health effects occuring. In consequence, when deriving an air quality standard for PM_{10} and $PM_{2.5}$ using these relationships, it has to be decided which curve should be used with due consideration to confidence intervals, and the risk has to be fixed. This is a new situation with respect to the derivation of an air quality standard from an air quality value, in which a risk is assumed without explicitly stating it.

The following observations should be kept in mind when using these graphs:

- For PM_{10} or $PM_{2.5}$ the graphs should not be used for concentrations below 20 or $10\mu g/m^3$ respectively, or above 200 or $100\mu g/m^3$ respectively. This is due to the fact that mean 24-hour concentrations below or above the quoted values could not be used for the risk assessment, and the curves presented in Figures 4.1 to 4.3 would present unvalidated extrapolations beyond the range of observed results.
- There is a fundamental difference between the guidelines for PM_{10} or $PM_{2.5}$ and the guideline value for respirable particulate matter of $70\mu g/m^3$ that was derived in the WHO air quality guidelines for Europe (WHO/EURO, 1987). The guidelines for PM_{10} and $PM_{2.5}$ are relationships between the percentage change in some health endpoint and the PM concentration. The guideline value for respirable PM (WHO/EURO, 1987) was a fixed value based upon the knowledge established in the epidemiological literature. Due to not finding a threshold for the onset of health effects caused by PM, a safe level could not be fixed for this compound.

The AMIS, a programme set up by WHO as a successor to the UNEP/WHO Global Environmental Monitoring System (GEMS/AIR) programme, provides valuable information on air pollutant monitoring and management in major cities and megacities (WHO, 1997a, 1998a, 2001). AMIS is a set of databases that were developed by WHO under the umbrella of the Healthy Cities Programme. The objective of AMIS is to transfer information on air quality management (air quality management instruments used in cities, ambient air pollutant concentrations, health effects, air quality standards, rapid emission assessment tools and global, regional and national estimates of the burden of disease due to air pollution) between countries and cities. In this context, AMIS

Table 4.1 *WHO air quality guidelines for 'classical' compounds*

Compound	Average ambient air concentration [$\mu g/m^3$]	Health endpoint	Observed effect level [$\mu g/m^3$]	Uncertainty factor	Guideline value [$\mu g/m^3$]	Averaging time
Carbon monoxide	500–7000	Critical level of COHb < 2.5%	n/a	n/a	100,000 60,000 30,000 10,000	15 minutes 30 minutes 1 hour 8 hours
Lead	0.01–2	Critical level of lead in blood <25μg lead per litre	n/a	n/a	0.5	1 year
Nitrogen dioxide	10–150	Slight changes in lung function in asthmatics	365–565	0.5	200 40	1 hour 1 year
Ozone	10–100	Respiratory function responses	n/a	n/a	120	8 hours
Sulphur dioxide	5–400	Changes in lung function in asthmatics Exacerbations of respiratory symptoms in sensitive individuals	1000 250 100	2 2 2	500 125 50	10 minutes 24 hours 1 year

Notes: COHb = carboxyhaemoglobin.
Average ambient air concentration level: Arithmetic mean or range of observed ambient air concentrations in urban areas.
Observed effect level: the lowest level at which no (adverse) effect was observed or the lowest level at which an adverse effect was observed.
Uncertainty factor: factor by which an observed or estimated toxic concentration or dose is divided to arrive at a guideline value that is considered safe. Such a factor allows for a variety of uncertainties, for example, about possibly undetected effects on particularly sensitive members of the population, synergistic effects and the adequacy of existing data. Traditionally, the uncertainty factor has been used to allow for uncertainties in extrapolation from animals to humans and from a small group of individuals to a large population.

Table 4.2 *WHO air quality guidelines for non-carcinogenic compounds*

Compound	Average ambient air concentration [μg/m³]	Health endpoint	Observed effect level [mg/m³]	Uncertainty factor	Guideline value [μg/m³]	Averaging time	Source
Acetaldehyde	5	Irritancy in humans	45 (NOEL)	20	2,000	24 hours	WHO, 1995b
		Carcinogenicity-related irritation in rats	275 (NOEL)	1000	300	1 year	WHO, 1995b
Acrolein	15	Eye irritation in humans	130	2.5	50	30 minutes	WHO, 1992
Acrylic acid	No data	Nasal lesions in mice	15 (LOAEL)	50	54	1 year	WHO, 1997c
Cadmium	$(0.1–20) \times 10^{-3}$	Renal effects in the population	n/a	n/a	5×10^{-3}	1 year	WHO/EURO, 2000
Carbon disulphide	10–1500	Functional central nervous system	10 (LOAEL)	100	100	24 hours	WHO/EURO, 1987
		Odour annoyance (odour threshold)	n/a	n/a	20	30 minutes	WHO/EURO, 1987
Chloroform	0.3–110	Hepatoxicity in beagles	from TDI	1000	15	24 hours	WHO, 1994a
1,2-Dichloroethane	0.2–6	Inhalation in animals	700 (LOAEL)	1000	700	24 hours	WHO/EURO, 1987
Dichloromethane	< 5	COHb formation in normal subjects	n/a	n/a	3,000	24 hours	WHO/EURO, 2000
Diesel exhaust	1.0–10.0	Chronic alveolar inflammation in humans	0.139 (NOAEL)	25	5.6	1 year	WHO, 1996a
		Chronic alveolar inflammation in rats	0.23 (NOAEL)	100	2.3	1 year	WHO, 1996a
Di-n-butyl Phthalate	$(3–80) \times 10^{-3}$	Developmental/reproductive toxicity	from ADI	1000	14	24 hours	WHO, 1997d
Ethylbenzene	1–100	Biological significance criteria in animals	2150 (NOEL)	100	22,000	1 week	WHO, 1996b
Fluorides	0.5–3	Effects on livestock	n/a	n/a	1	1 year	WHO, 1994b
Formaldehyde	$(1–20) \times 10^{-3}$	Nose, throat irritation in humans	0.1 (NOAEL)	n/a	0.1	30 minutes	WHO/EURO, 2000

Substance	Average ambient air concentration	Effect	Observed effect level	Uncertainty factor	Guideline value	Averaging time	Source
Hydrogen sulphide	0.15	Eye irritation in humans	15 (LOAEL)	100	150	24 hours	WHO/EURO, 1987
		Odour annoyance (odour threshold)	n/a	n/a	7	30 minutes	WHO/EURO, 1987
Manganese	0.01–0.07	Neurotoxic effects in workers	0.03 (NOAEL)	200	0.15	1 year	WHO/EURO, 2000
Mercury, inorganic	$(2$–$10) \times 10^{-3}$	Renal tubular effects in humans	0.02 (LOAEL)	20	1	1 year	WHO/EURO, 2000
Styrene	1.0–20.0	Neurological effects in workers	107 (LOAEL)	400	260	1 week	WHO/EURO, 2000
		Odour annoyance (odour threshold)	n/a	n/a	70	30 minutes	WHO/EURO, 2000
Tetrachloroethylene	1–5	Kidney effects in workers	102 (LOAEL)	400	250	24 hours	WHO/EURO, 2000
		Odour annoyance (odour threshold)	n/a	n/a	8000	30 minutes	WHO/EURO, 1987
Toluene	5–150	Effects on CNS in workers	332 (LOAEL)	1260	260	1 week	WHO/EURO, 2000
		Odour annoyance (odour threshold)	n/a	n/a	1000	30 minutes	WHO/EURO, 1987
Vanadium	0.05–0.2	Respiratory effects in workers	0.02 (LOAEL)	20	1	24 hours	WHO/EURO, 1987
Xylenes	1–100	Neurotoxicity in rats	870 (LOAEL)	1000	870	1 year	WHO, 1997e
		CNS effects in human volunteers	304 (NOAEL)	60	4800	24 hours	WHO, 1997e
		Odour annoyance (odour threshold)	n/a	n/a	4400	30 minutes	WHO, 1997e

Notes: COHb = carboxyhaemoglobin.

Average ambient air concentration level: arithmetic mean or range of observed ambient air concentrations in urban areas.

Observed effect level: the lowest level at which a low (adverse) effect was observed (NOEL, NOAEL) or the lowest level at which an adverse effect was observed (LOAEL).

Uncertainty factor: factor by which an observed or estimated toxic concentration or dose is divided to arrive at a guideline value that is considered safe. Such a factor allows for a variety of uncertainties, for example, about possibly undetected effects on particularly sensitive members of the population, synergistic effects and the adequacy of existing data. Traditionally, the uncertainty factor has been used to allow for uncertainties in extrapolation from animals to humans and from a small group of individuals to a large population.

ADI: maximum amount of a substance to which a subject may be exposed daily over its lifetime without appreciable health risk.

TDI: estimate of the amount of a substance that can be ingested or absorbed over a period of a day without appreciable health risk.

Table 4.3 *WHO air quality guidelines for carcinogenic compounds*

Compound	Average ambient air concentration [µg/m³]	Health endpoint	Unit risk [µg/m³]⁻¹	IARC classification	Source
Acetaldehyde	5	Nasal tumours in rats	$(1.5-9) \times 10^{-7}$	2B	WHO, 1995b
Acrylonitrile	0.01–10	Lung cancer in workers	2×10^{-5}	2A	WHO/EURO, 1987
Arsenic	$(1-30) \times 10$-3	Lung cancer in exposed humans	1.5×10^{-3}	1	WHO/EURO, 2000
Benzene	5.0–20.0	Leukaemia in exposed workers	6×10^{-6}	1	WHO/EURO, 2000
Chromium VI	$(5-200) \times 10$-3	Lung cancer in exposed workers	4×10^{-2}	1	WHO/EURO, 2000
Diesel exhaust	1.0–10.0	Lung cancer in rats	$(1.6-7.1) \times 10^{-5}$		WHO, 1996a
Nickel	1–180	Lung cancer in exposed humans	3.8×10^{-4}	1	WHO/EURO, 2000
PAH (BaP)	$(1-10) \times 10$-3	Lung cancer in exposed humans	8.7×10^{-5}	2A	WHO/EURO, 2000
Trichloroethylene	1–10	Cell tumours in testes of rats	4.3×10^{-7}	2A	WHO/EURO, 2000
Vinylchloride	0.1–10	Haemangiosarcoma in exposed workers / Liver cancer in exposed workers	1×10^{-6}	1	WHO/EURO, 1987
Fibres	[fibres/l]		[fibres/l]−1		
MMVF (RCF)	$2-2 \times 10^{3}$	Mesotheliomas in animal inhalation	1×10^{-6} $[Bq/m^3]$ $[Bq/m^3]^{-1}$	2B	WHO/EURO, 2000
Radon	100	Lung cancer in residentials	$(3-6) \times 10^{-5}$	1	WHO/EURO, 2000

Notes: Bq/m³: Becquerels per cubic metre
Fibres/l: fibres per litre.
PAH: polycyclic aromatic hydrocarbons.
BaP: benzo (a) pyrene.
MMVF: manmade vitreous fibres.
RCF: refractory ceramic fibres.
IARC: International Agency for Research on Cancer.
Average ambient air concentration level: arithmetic mean or range of observed ambient air concentrations in urban areas.
Unit risk: the additional lifetime cancer risk occurring in a hypothetical population in which all individuals are exposed continuously from birth throughout their lifetimes to a concentration of 1µg/m³ of the agent in the air they breathe.
IARC classification: IARC classifies chemicals for carcinogenicity in the following way: Group 1 = proven human carcinogens; Group 2 = probable human carcinogens; Group 2A = probable human carcinogens according to higher degree of evidence; Group 2B = probable human carcinogens according to lower degree of evidence; Group 3 = unclassified chemicals.

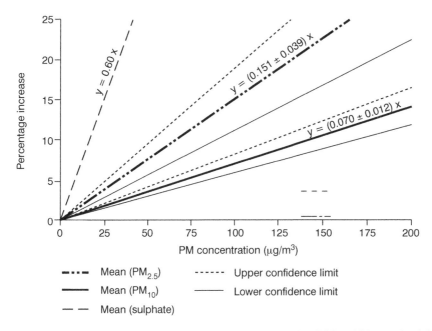

Figure 4.1 *Percentage increase in daily mortality assigned to PM_{10}, $PM_{2.5}$ and sulphates*

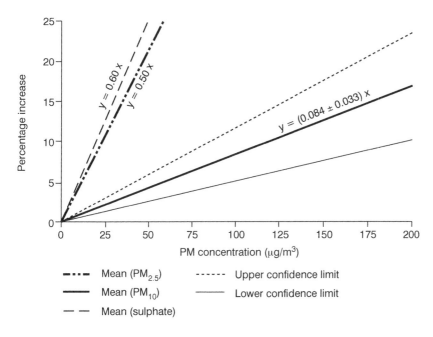

Figure 4.2 *Percentage change in hospital admissions assigned to PM_{10}, $PM_{2.5}$ and sulphates*

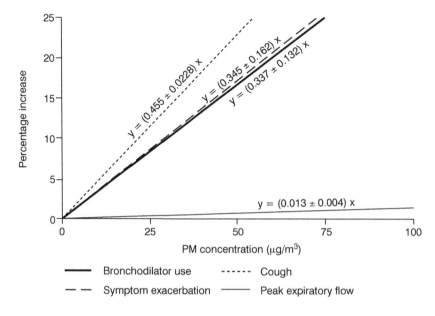

Figure 4.3 *Change in health endpoints in relation to PM$_{10}$ concentrations*

acts as a global air quality information exchange system. AMIS programme activity areas include:

- coordinating databases with information on air quality issues in major cities and megacities;
- acting as an information broker between countries;
- providing and distributing technical documents on air quality and health;
- publishing and distributing trend reviews on air pollutant concentrations; and
- organizing training courses on air quality and health.

AMIS provides a set of user-friendly Microsoft Access-based databases. A core database contains summary statistics of air pollution data such as annual means, 95-percentiles and the number of days on which WHO guidelines are exceeded. Any compound for which WHO air quality guidelines exist can be entered into the open-ended database. Data handling is easy and data validation can be assured with relatively limited means. In the present version, data (mostly from 1986 to 1998) from about 150 cities in 45 countries are represented (WHO, 2001). Another AMIS database covers the air pollution management capabilities and procedures of cities. Databases on the use and accessibility of dispersion models, control actions, health effects and the magnitudes of their respective costs are also planned.

The following discussion covers legal aspects, exposure–response relationships, the characterization of exposure, the assessment and acceptability of risks, application of cost–benefit analysis (CBA) and the enforcement of air quality standards through the instrument of clean air implementation plans.

USE OF WHO GUIDELINES FOR AIR QUALITY IN LOCAL AIR QUALITY MANAGEMENT

For air quality management to be effective, goals, policies, strategies and tactics have to be defined. Goals for air quality management can include the elimination or reduction to acceptable levels of ambient air pollutant concentrations or the avoidance of adverse effects on humans and other receptors. Policies for air quality management encompass clean air acts, environmental impact assessments, air quality standards, clean air implementation plans and cost–benefit comparisons. Strategies for air quality management refer to command-and-control procedures and/or the application of market mechanisms. The tactical instruments of air quality management are inventories, dispersion modelling, monitoring and comparison with standards.

A framework for a political, regulatory and administrative approach is required to guarantee a consistent and transparent derivation of air quality standards and to ensure a basis for decisions on risk-reducing measures and abatement strategies. In such a framework, legal aspects, adverse effects on health, the population at risk, exposure–response relationships, exposure characterization, risk assessment, the acceptability of risk, CBA and stakeholder contribution in standard setting have to be included.

Legal aspects

A legislative framework usually provides the basis for policies in the decision-making process of setting air quality standards at the municipal, regional, national or supranational level. The setting of standards strongly depends on the risk management strategy adopted, which, in turn, is influenced by country-specific socio-political and economic considerations and/or international agreements. Legislation and air quality standards vary from country to country, but in general, the WHO guidelines for air quality and the information provided by AMIS can provide guidance on how to consider the following issues in developing countries:

*   **Identification of the pollutants to be considered:** Provided the types of sources are known, the guidelines and the rapid assessment procedures of AMIS can identify the most important sources and estimate their emissions.
*   **Existing background concentrations of air pollutants:** The knowledge on global concentrations from the AMIS database on air pollutant concentrations and the WMO Global Atmospheric Watch can serve to estimate background concentrations. The Decision Support System for Industrial Pollution Control (DSS IPC) is a useful and user-friendly instrument to estimate concentrations on the basis of initial emissions estimates and simple dispersion models.

- **Applicable monitoring methodology and its quality assurance:** The most appropriate and least-cost means for ground-based monitoring can be selected on the basis of the AMIS-GEMS/AIR Methodology Handbook Review Series (UNEP/WHO, 1994a, 1994b, 1994c, 1994d). In these publications WHO gives simple advice on monitoring, siting and quality assurance when existing information and means are minimal. These publications are being updated and revised (WHO, 2002). Publications from other agencies also provide insight into monitoring strategies (McGinlay et al, 1996; Aggarwal and Gopal, 1996; Lahmann, 1997; Martinez and Romieu, 1997).
- **The numerical value of the standards for the various pollutants or the decision-making process:** Air quality standards may be based on WHO air quality guidelines, but other aspects, such as technological feasibility, costs of compliance, prevailing exposure levels and social and economic cultural conditions are also relevant to the standard setting procedure and the design of appropriate emission abatement measures. Several air quality standards may be set, eg effect-oriented standards as a long term goal and less stringent standards to be achieved within shorter time intervals. As a consequence, air quality standards differ widely from country to country (WHO, 1998b). The guidelines for air quality enable country-specific air quality standards to be derived based on existing or estimated concentrations. The cost of control estimates and the efficiency of controls can be assessed using the DSS IPC (WHO, 1993b, 1995a).
- **Emission control measures and emission standards:** Given the types of sources and estimations of their emissions via the rapid assessment method and their spatial distribution, the DSS IPC can serve to simulate the efficiency of control measures and help to set appropriate emission standards for the main sources (WHO/PAHO/WB, 1995).
- **Identification and selection of adverse effects on public health and the environment to be avoided:** Health effects range from death and acute illness, through chronic and lingering diseases and minor and temporary ailments, to temporary physiological or psychological changes. The guidelines advise on the more serious adverse effects of air pollutants. Health effects that are either temporary or reversible, or involve biochemical or functional changes with uncertain clinical significance, need not be considered in the first step of deriving a standard in developing countries. Judgements as to adversity of health effects may differ between countries because of, for example, different cultural backgrounds and different levels of health status.
- **Identification of the population to be protected from adverse effects on health:** The most sensitive sub-groups of the population are identified in the guidelines as infants, pregnant women, disabled persons and the elderly. Other groups may be judged to be at higher risk due to enhanced exposure (outdoor workers, athletes and children). The sensitive groups in a population may vary across countries due to differences in medical care, nutritional status, lifestyle and/or prevailing genetic factors, or due to the existence of endemic diseases or the prevalence of debilitating diseases.

The air quality guidelines have been set with respect to the sub-groups more sensitive to air pollution. Setting standards on the basis of the guidelines and considering the consequence of uncertainty provide at least some protection for these sub-populations.

Air quality standards strongly influence the implementation of air pollution control policies. In many countries, the exceeding of standards is linked to an obligation to develop action plans at the municipal, regional or national level to abate air pollution (clean air implementation plans).

Exposure–response relationships

In general, there is limited information available on exposure–response relationships for inorganic and organic pollutants, especially at low exposures. The revised air quality guidelines for Europe provide exposure–response relationships for a number of pollutants including detailed tables of the relationships for particulate matter (PM) and ozone. For PM_{10} and $PM_{2.5}$ the changes of various health endpoints such as daily mortality and hospital admissions with each $10\mu g/m^3$ increase in concentrations are quantified.

If it can be assumed that these relationships apply across the entire range of concentrations between 0 and $200\mu g/m^3$, then the available data imply that there are linear relationships between various health endpoints and PM concentrations. For carcinogenic compounds, the quantitative assessment of the unit risks provides an approximate estimate of responses at different concentrations. These relationships, which are extensively discussed in the Guidelines for Air Quality, give guidance to decision-makers to determine the acceptable risk for the population exposure to particulate matter and to carcinogenic compounds and set the corresponding concentrations as standards.

Exposure characterization

Exposure to air pollution is not only determined by ambient air pollutant concentrations. In deriving air quality standards that protect against adverse health impacts, the size of the population at risk (ie exposed to enhanced air pollutant concentrations) is an important factor to consider. The total exposure of people also depends on the time people spend in the various environments: outdoor, indoor, workplace, in-vehicle and other. Exposure also depends on the various routes of intake and absorption of pollutants in the human body: air, water, food and tobacco smoking. Therefore, it should be kept in mind that there is a weak relationship between pollutant concentrations and personal exposures. An example of this weak relationship is provided by indoor air pollution, when biomass fuels are used for heating and cooking. However, in developing countries, ambient air concentrations are at present the only readily available surrogate for estimating personal exposures.

Risk assessment

WHO air quality guidelines are based on health or ecological risk models. These models provide a tool that is increasingly used to inform policy-makers about some of the possible consequences of air pollutants at different pollutant levels, which correspond to various options for standards. Using this information, the policy-maker is able to perform a regulatory risk assessment of air pollution-induced effects. Regulatory risk assessment in air pollution management includes the following steps: hazard identification, development of exposure–response relationships, exposure analysis and quantitative risk estimation. The first step, hazard identification – and, to some extent, the second step, exposure–response relationships – have already been provided in the air quality guidelines. The third step, exposure analysis, may predict changes in exposure associated with reductions in emissions from a specific source or group of sources under different control options. The final step in regulatory risk assessment, risk analysis, refers to the quantitative estimation of the risk of health effects in the exposed population (eg the number of individuals who may be affected). Examples for such estimates were given by Hong (1995), Ostro (1996), Schwela (1996), Murray and Lopez (1997) and Schwela (1998). Regulatory risk assessments are likely to result in different risk estimates across countries and economic regions owing to differences in exposure patterns and in the size and characteristics of sensitive groups. In addition, differences in the legislation and availability of information necessary to undertake quantitative risk assessments may affect the results.

Acceptability of risk

In the absence of thresholds for the onset of health effects – as in the cases of fine and ultrafine particulate matter and carcinogenic compounds – the selection of an air quality standard that provides adequate protection of public health requires the regulator to determine an acceptable risk for the population. Acceptability of the risks, and therefore the standards selected, will depend on the expected incidence and severity of the potential effects, the size of the population at risk, and the degree of scientific uncertainty that the effects will occur at any given level of air pollution. For example, if a suspected but uncertain health effect is severe and the size of the population at risk is large, a more cautious approach would be appropriate than if the effect were less troubling or if the population were smaller.

The acceptability of risk may vary among countries because of differences in social norms, degree of risk aversion and perception in the general population and various stakeholders. Risk acceptability is also influenced by how the risks associated with air pollution compare with risks from other pollution sources or human activities (de Koning, 1987).

Cost–benefit analysis

Two different approaches for decisions can be applied in the derivation of air quality standards from air quality guidelines. In the first approach, decisions are based purely on health, cultural and environmental consequences with little attention to economic efficiency. The objective of this approach is to reduce the risk of adverse effects to a socially acceptable level. The second approach is based on a formal cost-effectiveness or CBA, the objective being to identify the control action that achieves greatest net economic benefit or is the most economically efficient. The development of air quality standards should take account of both extremes. CBA is a highly inter-disciplinary task and, if appropriately applied and not used as the sole and overriding determinant of decisions, can be a legitimate and useful way to provide information for risk managers making decisions that will affect human health and the environment.

The WHO guidelines for air quality describe in some detail the individual steps of a CBA and give advice on which information is needed to undertake CBA. In developed countries, at least part of this information can be made available but, in most developing countries, comprehensive CBA procedures can only be applied in the long term. It would be useful for developing countries to collect data on the use of medication, number of hospital admissions, outpatient visits or days of labour lost and relate them to air pollution. This procedure would at least give some indication of the potential magnitude of the benefits of air pollution control (WHO, 1998b).

Review of standard setting

The setting of standards should encompass a process involving stakeholders (industry, local authorities, non-governmental organizations and the general public) that assures – as far as possible – social equity or fairness to all the parties involved. It should also provide sufficient information to guarantee understanding by stakeholders of the scientific and economic consequences. The earlier stakeholders are involved, the more likely is their cooperation. Transparency in moving from air quality guidelines to air quality standards helps to increase public acceptance of necessary measures. Raising public awareness of air pollution-induced health and environmental effects (changing of risk perception) serves to obtain public support for the necessary control action, eg with respect to vehicular emissions. Information provided to the public with regard to air quality during pollution episodes and the risks entailed lead to a better understanding of the issue (risk communication).

Air quality standards should be reviewed and revised regularly as new scientific evidence on the effects on public health and the environment emerges.

ENFORCEMENT OF AIR QUALITY STANDARDS: CLEAN AIR IMPLEMENTATION PLANS

The enforcement of air quality standards ensures that actions are taken to control polluting sources in order to comply with the standards. The instruments used to achieve this goal are clean air implementation plans (CAIPs). The outline of such a plan is usually defined in regulatory policies and strategies. CAIPs were implemented in several developed countries during the 1970s and 1980s. At that time the air pollutant situation was characterized by a multitude of different types of sources leading to an extremely difficult causal assessment of public health risks with respect to single sources or groups of sources. As a consequence, and on the basis of the 'polluter pays' principle, sophisticated tools were developed to assess the pollution sources, air pollutant concentrations, health and environmental effects and control measures. The tools also made a causal link between emissions, the air pollution situation and the efficiency of the necessary control measures. The CAIP has proved to be a most efficient instrument for air pollution abatement in developed countries (Schwela and Köth-Jahr, 1994; WHO, 1997b).

In developing countries, the air pollution situation is often characterized by a multitude of sources of few types, and sometimes few sources. Using the experience obtained in developed countries, the control action to be taken is often very clear. As a consequence, a lower intensity of monitoring would be sufficient, and dispersion models could help to simulate spatial distributions of concentrations if only limited useful monitoring data are available. Only simplified CAIPs would have to be developed for cities in developing countries or countries in transition. The main polluters at present in many cities in the developing world are old vehicles and some industrial sources such as power plants, brick kilns and cement factories.

In such situations, a simplified CAIP could include:

- a rapid assessment of the most important sources (Economopoulos 1993a, 1993b; WHO, 1995a);
- a minimal set of air pollutant concentration monitors (UNEP/WHO, 1994a, 1994c, 1994d);
- simulation of the spatial distribution of air pollutant concentrations using simple dispersion models (WHO/PAHO/WB, 1995);
- comparison with air quality standards;
- control measures and their costs (WHO/PAHO/WB, 1995); and
- transportation and land use planning.

Examples of successful simplified CAIPs in developing countries are provided in a recent report on air quality management capabilities in 20 major cities (UNEP/WHO/MARC, 1996) and on the third edition of the AMIS CD-ROM for 70 cities (WHO, 2001).

URBAN AIR QUALITY MANAGEMENT IN EUROPE

European directives are increasingly influencing the management of air quality in EU Member States. The objective of the Framework Directive 96/62/EC on ambient air quality assessment and management (CEC, 1996) is to outline a common strategy to:

- establish emissions limits to improve ambient air quality;
- assess ambient air quality in the EU on the basis of common methods and criteria;

Table 4.4 *EU limit values for outdoor air quality (health protection)*

Pollutant	Limit value [$\mu g/m^3$]	Averaging period	Number of exceedences [times]	To be implemented by	Directive
SO_2	350	1 hr	<25	1.1.2005	CEC, 1999
	125	24 hrs	<4	1.1.2005	CEC, 1999
NO_2	200	1 hr	<19	1.1.2010	CEC, 1999
	40	1 yr	0	1.1.2010	CEC, 1999
PM_{10}*	50	24 hrs	<36	1.1.2005	CEC, 1999
	40	1 yr	0	1.1.2005	CEC, 1999
Lead	0.5	1 yr	0	1.1.2005	CEC, 1999
O_3	120	8 hrs	<26 days	2010	EC, 2000
CO	10,000	8 hrs	0	1.1.2010	CEC, 2000
Benzene	5	1 yr	0	1.1.2010	CEC, 2000

Note: *These limits should be reached by 2005; the setting of more stringent limit values will depend on a review in 2003–2004.

- ensure adequate information is made available to the public; and
- maintain ambient air quality where it is good and improve it in other cases.

The Framework Directive (CEC, 1996) considers air quality standards for already regulated atmospheric pollutants (SO_2, NO_2, PM, lead and O_3) and for benzene, carbon monoxide, polycyclic aromatic hydrocarbons, cadmium, arsenic, nickel and mercury. The Framework Directive and its daughter directives (CEC, 1996, 1999, 2000) include a timetable for the implementation of air quality standards for 12 individual pollutants. The objectives of the daughter directives are to harmonize monitoring strategies, measuring methods, calibration and quality assessment methods to achieve comparable measurements throughout the EU and good information to the public. Table 4.4 presents the limit values for different pollutants covered by the Framework and daughter directives.

The European Union (EU), in its programme for Clean Air for Europe (CAFE) has developed a thematic strategy for improving air quality in Europe. This strategy is based on four elements (EC, 2001):

1 developing emission limits for ambient air quality;
2 combating the effects of transboundary air pollution;
3 identifying cost-effective reductions in targeted areas through integrated programmes; and
4 introducing specific measures to limit emissions.

The main elements of the programme are:

- to review the implementation of air quality directives and the effectiveness of air quality programmes in the Member States; and

- to improve the monitoring of air quality and the provision of information to the public, including the use of indicators, priorities for further action, the review and updating of air quality standards and national emission ceilings and the development of better systems for gathering information, modelling and forecasting.

A review of good practice in European urban air quality management (UAQM) was undertaken by Eurocities, which is an association of European metropolitan cities. The association represents 90 cities from 26 European countries and 17 associated members and, through its thematic sub-networks, many more large, medium sized and small cities in Europe and beyond. The network aims to improve the quality of life of the 80 per cent of Europeans living in cities and urban areas by influencing the European agenda, and promoting the exchange of experience and best practice between city governments. The review addressed UAQM issues in six European cities: Bologna (Italy), Bratislava (Slovakia), Delft (The Netherlands), Helsinki (Finland), Lisbon (Portugal) and Sheffield (UK). The six countries examined national and European legislation to improve urban air quality. However, this was in addition to a variety of initiatives such as Local Agenda 21, urban CO_2 reduction, public transport provision and public awareness campaigns.

One main point highlighted in the Eurocities study was that local air quality management is the most effective way of addressing urban air quality problems. This involves cooperation with city authorities and industry, commerce, public transport providers and the public.

All six European cities recognized road traffic emissions as being the single most important and complex issue for air quality management to address. The Eurocities study recommends that:

- The inappropriate use of motor vehicles should be tackled by city authorities working together with other cities and countries to develop affordable, attractive and accessible alternatives to the private car.
- Business travel plans should be used to address commuter journeys as they can bring about a combination of improvements and cost savings for organizations as well as many less tangible benefits for staff and society as a whole.
- Decisions on appropriate use of transport should be made at the local level in consultation with a wide range of stakeholders, eg planners, developers and the public.
- Local Agenda 21 should be a common thread that runs through all the measures that aim to reduce vehicle emissions.
- A long term commitment to public transport, with adequate investment, is important for the cities of the future.
- Air quality management should be part of a wider strategy and action for sustainable development.
- Policies of transportation, land use, planning, economic regeneration and air quality must be integrated to ensure that separate policies and actions are working in harmony to achieve common goals.

All the cities involved in the study believe that simply supplying air quality measurements to the public is no longer sufficient or acceptable. Information on air quality should be used to instigate awareness and education campaigns. These can play a major role in changing stakeholders' perceptions of air quality and encouraging them to contribute to, and be involved in, improving air quality. The Eurocities study concluded that there is:

> *a need for a flow of information on air quality management between cities and countries, so that a unified approach to meeting the needs of the Air Quality Framework Directive can be achieved. Examples have been cited which outline the need for coordination and cooperation within agencies. One of the main aspects of successful air quality management will be inter- and intra-cooperation. Once this has been achieved, a coherent planning stage can be instigated. A planning stage, which is clear and accessible to those outside the local authority must be produced. This in turn will be the basis for the essential next step – involving the wider community in air quality management.* (Eurocities, 1996)

The Eurocities study was followed by an Air Action project entitled *Achieving Change Locally*, the final report of the study (Eurocities, 2000). The aim of the project was to develop local air quality action plans in collaboration with business partners with an emphasis on land use and transport issues.

In a major review prepared under the Convention on Long-range Transboundary Air Pollution, the UN Economic Commission for Europe (UN/ECE) reviewed the strategies and policies for air pollution abatement (UN/ECE 1999). In the report, national strategies and policies with respect to air pollution abatement were discussed and compared with each other. These included the legislative and regulatory framework for integrating air pollution policy and energy, transport, economic and other policy areas. National measures considered included regulatory measures such as air quality and emission standards, fuel quality standards and deposition standards. Economic instruments such as taxes, emission trading and subsidies, and measures related to emission control technology were the cornerstones of national policy measures that are applied in most countries of the European region. Activities, which take place under the Convention, are aimed at harmonizing the legal framework among countries and increasing the exchange of control technology. While the scope of this report refers to the Convention, many ideas developed with respect to the Convention also apply to local air quality management.

CONCLUSIONS

This chapter has presented a simplified procedure for setting air quality standards from guidelines and implementing action plans for air pollution abatement in developing countries. Issues such as rapid emissions assessment and the use of dispersion modelling as a surrogate for extensive air pollutant concentration monitoring and the testing of local air pollutant concentrations against air quality standards for local ambient air quality management have been discussed. Air quality standards are often based on WHO air quality guidelines. In moving from air quality guidelines to air quality standards, several factors have to be considered including the political, regulatory and administrative approaches to the control of air pollution. The WHO guidelines for air quality and AMIS provide guidance in achieving effective air quality management in developing countries. This guidance is well in line with recent developments in Europe within the EU CAFE programme.

References

Aggarwal, A L and Gopal, S K (eds) (1996) *Ambient Air Quality Monitoring Networks: Considerations for Developing Countries*, World Health Organization Regional Office for South-East Asia, New Delhi

CEC (1996) Council Directive 96/62/EC of 27 September on ambient air quality assessment and management, Official Journal L 296, 21/11/1996, pp55–63, Brussels

CEC (1999) Council Directive 1999/30/EC of 22 April relating to limit values for sulphur dioxide, nitrogen dioxide and oxides of nitrogen, particulate matter and lead in ambient air, Official Journal L 163, 29/06/1999, pp41–60

CEC (2000) Directive 2000/69/EC of the European Parliament and of the Council of 16 November relating to limit values for benzene and carbon monoxide in ambient air, Official Journal, L 313, 13/12/2000, p12

EC (2000) Amendment proposal for a Directive of the European Parliament and of the Council relating to ozone in ambient air, COM (2000) 613 final, 2.10.2000, European Commission, Brussels

EC (2001) 'The Clean Air For Europe (CAFE) Programme: towards a thematic strategy for air quality', Communication from the Commission, COM (2001) 245 final, 4.05.2001, European Commission, Brussels

Economopoulos, A (1993a) *Assessment of Sources of Air, Water and Land Pollution, Part One: Rapid Inventory Techniques in Environmental Pollution*, WHO/PEP/GETNET/93.1–A, World Health Organization, Geneva

Economopoulos, A (1993b) *Assessment of Sources of Air, Water and Land Pollution, Part Two: Approaches for Consideration in Formulating Environmental Control Strategies*, WHO/PEP/GETNET/93.1–B, World Health Organization, Geneva

Eurocities (1996) 'Good practice in european urban air quality management', www.eurocities.org

Eurocities (2000) 'The Air Action Project: achieving change locally', www.eurocities.org

Hong, C J (1995) *Global Burden of Diseases from Air Pollution* (unpublished)

de Koning, H W (ed) (1987) *Setting Environmental Standards: Guidelines for Decision-making*, World Health Organization, Geneva

Lahmann, E (ed) (1997) *Determination and Evaluation of Ambient Air Quality – Manual of Ambient Air Monitoring in Germany*, second revised edition, Federal Environmental Agency, Berlin

McGinlay, J, Vallance-Plews, J and Bower, J (eds) (1996) *Air Quality Monitoring: A Handbook for Local Authorities, AEA Technology*, AEA/RAMP/20029001/01, Atomic Energy Agency, Abingdon, UK

Martinez, A P and Romieu, I (eds) (1997) *Introducción al Monitoreo Atmosférico*, World Health Organization/Pan American Health Organization, Mexico DF, Mexico

Murray, C J L and Lopez, A D (eds) (1996) *The Global Burden of Disease*, Harvard School of Public Health, Harvard University Press, Cambridge, MA

Schwela, D H (1996) 'Exposure to environmental chemicals relevant for respiratory hypersensitivity: global aspects' in *Toxicology Letters*, vol 86, pp131–142

Schwela, D H (1998) *Health and Air Pollution – A Developing Country's Perspective*, keynote address at the 11th World Clean Air and Environment Congress, Durban, South Africa, 13–18 September

Schwela, D H (2000a) *The World Health Organization Guidelines for Air Quality, Part 1: Exposure–response Relationships and Air Quality Guidelines*, WHO, Geneva, pp29–34

Schwela, DH (2000b) *The World Health Organization Guidelines for Air Quality, Part 2: Air Quality Management and the Role of the Guidelines*, WHO, Geneva, pp23–27

Schwela, D H and Köth-Jahr, I (1994) *Leitfaden für die Aufstellung von Luftreinhalteplänen* (Guidelines for the Implementation of Clean Air Implementation Plans), Report No 4, Landesumweltamt Nordrhein Westfalen, Essen, Germany

UN/ECE (1999) *Strategies and Policies for Air Pollution Abatement,* ECE/EB.AIR/65, United Nations, New York and Geneva

UNEP/WHO (1994a) *GEMS/AIR Methodology Review Handbook Series, Volume 1: Quality Assurance in Urban Air Quality Monitoring*, United Nations Environment Programme, Nairobi/World Health Organization, Geneva

UNEP/WHO (1994b) *GEMS/AIR Methodology Review Handbook Series, Volume 2: Primary Standard Calibration Methods and Network Intercalibrations for Air Quality Monitoring,* United Nations Environment Programme, Nairobi/World Health Organization, Geneva

UNEP/WHO (1994c) *GEMS/AIR Methodology Review Handbook Series, Volume 3: Measurement of Suspended Particulate Matter in Ambient Air*, United Nations Environment Programme, Nairobi/World Health Organization, Geneva

UNEP/WHO (1994d) *GEMS/AIR Methodology Review Handbook Series, Volume 4: Passive and Active Sampling Methodologies for Measurement of Air Quality*, United Nations Environment Programme, Nairobi/World Health Organization, Geneva

UNEP/WHO/MARC (1996) *GEMS/AIR Air Quality Management and Assessment Capabilities in 20 Major Cities*, Environmental Assessment Report, United Nations Environment Programme, Nairobi/World Health Organization, Geneva/The Monitoring and Assessment Research Centre, London

WHO (1992) *Acrolein*, Environmental Health Criteria 127, World Health Organization, Geneva

WHO (1994a) *Chloroform*, Environmental Health Criteria 163, World Health Organization, Geneva

WHO (1994b) *Updating and Revision of the Air Quality Guidelines for Europe – Inorganic Air Pollutants*, EUR/ICP/EHAZ 94 05/MT04, World Health Organization Regional Office for Europe, Copenhagen

WHO (1995) *Acetaldehyde*, Environmental Health Criteria 167, World Health Organization, Geneva

WHO (1996a) *Diesel Fuel and Exhaust Emissions*, Environmental Health Criteria 171, World Health Organization, Geneva

WHO (1996b) *Ethylbenzene*, Environmental Health Criteria 186, World Health Organization, Geneva

WHO (1997a) *Healthy Cities Air Management Information System* (AMIS 1.0 CD ROM), World Health Organization, Geneva

WHO (1997b) *Health and Environment in Sustainable Development – Five Years after the Earth Summit*, World Health Organization, Geneva

WHO (1997c) *Acrylic Acid*, Environmental Health Criteria 191, World Health Organization, Geneva

WHO (1997d) *Di-n-Butyl Phthalate*, Environmental Health Criteria 189, World Health Organization, Geneva

WHO (1997e) *Xylenes*, Environmental Health Criteria 190, World Health Organization, Geneva

WHO (1998a) *Healthy Cities Air Management Information System* (AMIS 2.0 CD ROM), World Health Organization, Geneva

WHO (1998b) *Guidance for Setting Air Quality Standards*, Report of a WHO Working Group, Barcelona, Spain, 12–14 May, EUR/ICP/EHPM 02.01.02, WHO Regional Office for Europe, Copenhagen

WHO (2000) *Guidelines for Air Quality*, WHO/SDE/OEH/00.02, World Health Organization, Geneva, www.who.int/peh/

WHO (2001) *Air Management Information System* (AMIS 3.0 CD ROM), World Health Organization, Geneva

WHO (2002) *AMIS Handbook of Methodologies in Air Pollution Management*, World Health Organization, Geneva

WHO/EURO (1987) *Air Quality Guidelines for Europe*, WHO Regional Publications, European Series No 23, World Health Organization, Copenhagen

WHO/EURO (2000) *Air Quality Guidelines for Europe*, Second Edition, WHO Regional Publications, European Series, No 91, World Health Organization Regional Office for Europe, Copenhagen, www.who.dk/

WHO/PAHO/WB (1995) *Decision Support System for Industrial Pollution Control (DSS IPC)* (PC programme for the assessment of air emission inventories, liquid and solid waste inventories, estimation of pollution in air, water and soil), PAHO/World Bank, Washington, DC

5

Rapid Assessment of Air Pollution and Health: Making Optimal Use of Data for Policy- and Decision-making

Yasmin von Schirnding

ABSTRACT

In many countries throughout the world air pollution concentrations are increasing, yet information on the associated health effects is lacking. Decision-makers nevertheless need to set policies and control strategies, often on the basis of limited data. Many situations arise in which it may be necessary to conduct rapid appraisals of air pollution and associated health effects. For instance, there may be an air pollution episode resulting from a toxic spill or environmental disaster that demands a rapid response; there may be community concern about a potential air pollution risk from a polluting industry; there may be a sudden rise in hospital admissions for air pollution-associated respiratory illness; or there may be a need to make best available use of routinely available data in order to establish air pollution control priorities or plan services. This chapter discusses various approaches that can be used to conduct rapid appraisals, recognizing that the specific needs of any one particular situation will determine which method or mix of methods will be optimal. Assessment methods that rely on obtaining information at the level of the individual, as well as at the group level, are discussed. In addition, the chapter discusses the collection of aggregate and individual level data needed for rapid appraisals, with emphasis on exposure assessment techniques. As the relationship between air pollution and health effects is complex and will depend on the circumstances in any one setting, rapid appraisals should not be considered as one-off efforts but rather as part of an overall programme on air pollution health effects assessment and control.

INTRODUCTION

In developing countries throughout the world, especially in Latin America, Eastern Europe and Asia, air pollution concentrations are reaching significant levels, yet information on the associated health effects is lacking. As a consequence, there is frequently little basis for decision-makers to prioritize among alternative control strategies and policies in deciding which pollutants need to be controlled, in what way and to what extent.

The relationship between air pollution and health is complex, and will depend on a variety of factors and circumstances, all of which may vary from setting to setting and from one population group or area to another. Data and information availability, as well as capacity, will vary from setting to setting.

In one area there may be a limited air pollution monitoring network in place, whilst in another a source emissions inventory may have been compiled. In one setting there may be scanty health-related information available only from clinic records, whilst in a different setting sophisticated epidemiological studies may have been conducted on the health impact of air pollution. Not only may there be a lack of data on air pollution exposures or on health effects in a particular setting, but also it may be difficult to extrapolate results of studies from one setting to another.

Need for rapid appraisals

Decision-makers are often faced with the need to act on the basis of uncertain knowledge, and to make a rapid appraisal of the situation based on an optimal use of a variety of information and data sources, with a minimal amount of investment in sophisticated research studies or monitoring of air pollution health effects.

There may be a range of differing circumstances in which a rapid appraisal is necessary. There may be a need to establish priorities for air pollution control based on a situational analysis of the existing air pollutants in an area and associated health effects in the population; or there may be a spill of toxic substances that requires rapid assessment of the potential exposures and health effects. There may be concern in a particular community about the potential health effects of emissions from a factory, causing speculation about an increase in respiratory disorders in young children and the elderly.

There may be a sudden marked increase in the number of hospital admissions for asthma, which needs rapid assessment in terms of the potential role of air pollution. There may be an air pollution episode of widespread regional significance, such as the recent forest fires in South-East Asia, which demands immediate, rapid assessment and response. Each situation/problem is different, and will require its own rapid assessment approach and response mechanism.

Some situations may require an assessment of the current or immediate past situation regarding the impact of air pollution on health, whereas other situations may require some future forecasting of the impact or of a scenario-based impact of some anticipated future exposure (for example, impacts associated with alternative transport systems, energy policies or urban air pollution trends in developing countries).

In general, however, regardless of the precise circumstances for which the rapid assessment is needed, in setting and evaluating policies, standards and control strategies, and in planning for the provision of health services, consideration of a range of rapid assessment methods and approaches is often necessary.

RAPID EPIDEMIOLOGICAL ASSESSMENT

Environmental epidemiology

Epidemiology, the cornerstone of public health (Lilienfeld and Lilienfeld, 1980; Mausner and Kramer, 1985; Rothman, 1986; WHO, 1993a), is by definition concerned with the distribution and causes of diseases and health effects in human populations. Environmental epidemiology is that sub-specialty of epidemiology which is concerned more specifically with the environmental determinants of diseases and health effects, and in understanding the nature of the relationship between environmental exposures such as air pollution and ill-health in population groups (WHO, 1983; Goldsmith, 1986; von Schirnding, 1997). Epidemiological studies provide 'real world' evidence of associations between air pollution and health based on normal living conditions and exposure situations (WHO, 1996).

Environmental epidemiologists have been described as 'canaries' (used in bygone days to detect toxic concentrations of carbon monoxide in mines), who are capable of giving warning of impending environmental disaster. Fortunately, their fate is not to die, as the unfortunate canaries of the coal miners did, 'but to sing – to call out in clear tones the nature and type of impending health danger that threatens' (Goldsmith, 1988).

Development of rapid appraisal approaches

The US Academy of Sciences Advisory Committee on Health for Medical Research and Development first coined the term 'rapid epidemiological assessment' in 1981. It has been described as a collection of methods that provides health information more rapidly, simply and at a lower cost than standard methods of data collection, yet also yields reliable results for use primarily at the local level (Anker, 1991).

The intention is thus to generate quickly information that is as reliable as possible, while at the same time being accurate and useful. Whilst there is no such thing as a 'quick and dirty' method when it comes to obtaining valid information on the health effects of exposures in human populations, nevertheless it is indeed possible to modify and adapt conventional methods, techniques and approaches to make more appropriate use of data for decision-making in special circumstances.

Table 5.1 *Rapid epidemiological assessment characteristics*

- Rapid
- Simple
- Low-cost
- Minimal data requirements
- Aid in priority setting and planning
- Identify critical issues, problems, hotspots
- Minimal human resource requirements
- Results easily communicated and understood

Rapid epidemiological assessment (REA) represents a new approach to epidemiological research drawing on well known methods and stressing speed and simplicity, adaptation to local conditions and the need to obtain information promptly at a level of precision demanded by decision-makers. It is thus a response to the need for timely and accurate information on which to base decisions.

Many of the traditional epidemiological methods are not well suited to an environment in which there are extremely limited financial resources, and a lack of people skilled in data collection and analysis (Anker, 1991). Epidemiological sampling techniques generally aim to obtain representative samples of fairly large areas. This usually involves many resources and a lot of time, and frequently results are not fed back quickly enough to influence action or decision-making processes. Thus, there is a need to find alternatives to the traditional methods.

Considering the implications for government and industry of instituting better control measures and policies to regulate pollutants, it is essential for rapid appraisals of air pollution and health to be conducted in as rigorous and unbiased a way as possible. It is inevitable, however, that some statistical precision will be sacrificed for the sake of speed and simplicity. Thus, strengths and weaknesses of each method need to be made explicit. Rapid assessments should not be considered as one-off efforts, but rather as part of an ongoing process to be updated and developed over time.

In addition, it is important to realize that REA methods are frequently goal-oriented to services and community needs, and are not necessarily geared to answer more fundamental questions on the nature of relationships between health and exposures. REA methods can be used under a variety of conditions: for example, to evaluate routine environmental health service functioning, or even during emergencies or times of crisis, for example, to target at-risk populations in need of attention (Guha Sapir, 1991) (Table 5.1).

REA focuses on two aspects of epidemiology: sampling methods that reduce the time and resources required to collect and analyse data from individuals, and methods for the collection, organization, analysis and presentation of data at the community level (Anker, 1991). In all respects, an important aim is always to obtain information that will shed light on associations between exposures and health effects that are worthy of further investigation, and to minimize the chances of drawing the wrong conclusions based on spurious associations.

A variety of epidemiological methods can be used to assess the relationship between air pollutants and exposures, some of which are sophisticated and time-consuming (not considered here), whilst others can be adapted for use in a rapid appraisal situation depending on the particular circumstances in question.

Before considering some of the REA methods that one might use to obtain the necessary information on the relationship between air pollutants and health effects, it is important to appreciate some of the key distinguishing factors relating to health effects in relation to air pollution exposures, which will influence which methods to use in a particular setting as well as the interpretation of the data.

Characteristics of air pollution-related health effects

Despite the fact that there is now a wealth of information on the health effects of air pollutants (WHO, 1987; WHO, 1999a), there is still much uncertainty regarding the contribution of air pollutants, either directly or indirectly, or singly or in combination, to the health of people in differing circumstances.

The health effects of air pollution exposures may occur over short or long periods of time, they may be reversible or irreversible, they may increase or decrease in time, and they may be continuous or temporary. They may be acute, for example, following relatively soon after an exposure (often a single major dose of a substance, such as may occur by accident or due to a chemical spill for example), or they may be chronic, occurring as a result of cumulative exposure to complex mixes over long periods of time.

A long period of time may elapse between the initial exposure and the appearance of an adverse health effect. Dispersal of the population at risk over time and the long incubation period make it difficult to reconstruct exposures. Acute health effects are thus often easier to detect than chronic effects, which may be difficult to relate to exposure to specific hazards or sources.

A hierarchy of effects may occur, ranging from minor, temporary ailments through to acute illness to chronic disease, with relatively resistant and susceptible persons at either extreme of the distribution. Outcomes may include death, specific defined diseases (for example, lung cancer), disease categories (respiratory illnesses such as pneumonia, asthma, bronchitis), symptom complexes (cough, wheezing) and biochemical/physiological changes that may not necessarily result in symptoms (for example, elevated levels of zinc protoporphyrin resulting from lead exposure).

Infants and young children may be at particular risk, as they take in more of a contaminant relative to their size than do adults, and they have immature and therefore particularly vulnerable physiologies. The unborn foetus is particularly susceptible. Elderly people are also vulnerable from a physiological point of view (for example, they may be more susceptible to lung infections than younger people). The vulnerability of individuals (as opposed to groups) may vary, however, and a range of susceptibilities to hazardous substances may occur.

Table 5.2 *Some criteria for establishing causality*

• Strength of the association
• Specificity of the association
• Dose–response relationship
• Consistency of association
• Temporal relationship
• Biologic plausibility

Linking health outcomes to possible exposures is complex. Most health effects from air pollution are multifactorial insofar as the causal factors are concerned, and it may be difficult to determine the effects of one exposure in the light of the possible existence of simultaneous exposure to other factors. When dealing with low level exposures in particular, one may often be dealing with factors that play contributory rather than primary roles in the causation of an increased incidence of disease. The co-action of other factors may be needed for effects to occur.

Effects may be interactive, resulting in a reductive, additive or synergistic effect where the combined effect is greater than the sum of the individual effects. Combined effects may often arise from the influence of nutritional, dietary and other lifestyle factors such as smoking and alcohol intake.

Air pollution health assessments, regardless of the overall design, need to take into account issues such as confounding (interfering) factors and sources of bias, but some designs lend themselves better to dealing with such issues than others. Such designs are normally more sophisticated and time-consuming to conduct, however.

Normally it would not be possible to assess through rapid appraisal methods whether associations between air pollution and health effects were causal. Several criteria exist for assessing whether an association is likely to be causal or not (Bradford Hill, 1965; Griffith et al, 1993) (Table 5.2).

INDIVIDUAL LEVEL ASSESSMENT METHODS

In this section some methods for assessing health effects in relation to exposure are discussed (for a general discussion of methods see also Lilienfeld and Lilienfeld, 1980; WHO, 1983; Mausner and Kramer, 1985; Rothman, 1986; WHO, 1993a). These rely on information at the level of the individual as opposed to the group. Of importance is that in all studies sources of exposure are well identified, as well as populations at risk such as children and the elderly. The more the data are capable of being analysed in this way, the better the chances of developing control measures that are targeted at high risk population groups and areas.

Intervention study

Occasionally unusual circumstances may present themselves in which it may be feasible to conduct some form of a rapid intervention study, for example in a situation where a corrective action was tried out in reducing exposure, and it was possible to assess the health effects accordingly. An example would be the addition of scrubbers to an industrial plant, and the monitoring of exposures and health effects in the surrounding area, both prior to the intervention and subsequent to it. This would provide important data on the nature of potential air pollution-related health effects.

Cohort study

The situation could also arise in which it was possible to conduct a cohort (longitudinal or follow-up) study, which would involve following up defined population groups (exposed and unexposed respectively) over a certain period of time for a presumed health outcome, and measuring exposures (and other potential influencing factors) along the way. An example would be a study in which two comparable disease-free population groups, one exposed and one unexposed to indoor air pollution, were followed up over a period of time and the incidence of respiratory disorders in the two groups determined (see Armstrong and Campbell, 1991 for one example of this type of study design that might be adaptable).

In general, cohort studies allow for a more complete investigation of complex exposures or multiple outcomes, and can be used when detailed information becomes available about the exposure to characterize it effectively. They are, on the other hand, normally costly to conduct and involve a considerable amount of time and resources; therefore, they would not lend themselves easily to adaptation for a rapid appraisal, unless the health outcome of interest occurred relatively quickly, thus limiting the follow-up time necessary. One could also do such a study based on historical records, for example by assembling exposed and unexposed groups on the basis of hospital records and following them up to the present and determining disease status. This would involve a considerable time-saving.

Case control study

A case control study can yield important information fairly rapidly, if carefully conducted (Baltazar, 1991). This involves starting with a diseased population (ie, in this case a population with well documented air pollution-related health effects or symptomatology) and working backwards in time to determine or reconstruct the prior exposure. In pressing environmental problems, where the timeliness of findings may be important, the case control study, being relatively quick to conduct in many circumstances, may be appropriate. It can be rapid and efficient and provide reliable results when confounding factors (the influence of extraneous variables not under prime consideration for the purpose of the study at hand) are properly addressed.

Where it is possible to adequately classify cases and controls, this type of design can be used. An example would be a study that looked at exposure to indoor air pollution among children with pneumonia (cases) compared to children who were disease-free (controls) (see Robin et al, 1996 for one example of this type of study design which might be adaptable). An environmental 'outbreak' investigation would be a special application of this methodology, for example in a situation where there occurred a sudden release of a toxic substance or spill. Of critical importance in such studies is that the exposure information is accurately assessed. When relying on past exposure information, this may be difficult.

Cross-sectional study

A cross-sectional study is one in which a sample of the study population is investigated and the exposures and outcomes determined almost simultaneously in time. The information sought can be current (for example, relating to prevailing air pollution exposures) or past (relating to exposures to air pollution in the past). Whilst this type of design is of limited use in assessing the nature of potentially causal relationships due to the problem of the time sequence of events, it nevertheless has the advantage in that the relationship between several exposures and outcomes can be studied. These types of studies are often the first approaches used in assessing relationships.

An example would be a study in which a questionnaire is distributed to a cross-section of a community to obtain information on various potential exposures and health outcomes, such as respiratory health symptomatology and exposure to traffic, industry and indoor air pollution. Several communities or locations could be compared in this way. These studies provide a picture of the overall situation at a point in time, and can be rapid and inexpensive to conduct. If very large areas are to be sampled, areas within the region can be randomly selected, for example using multistage or stratified sampling techniques (see Pope and Dockery, 1996 for examples).

GROUP LEVEL ASSESSMENT METHODS

These methods rely on obtaining information at the level of the group as opposed to the individual, and therefore can be fairly rapidly conducted.

Ecological study

Ecological studies are weak in determining causality, as they involve measuring exposures and outcomes at the group level as opposed to the individual level, and making inferences about the relationship of exposures and outcomes in individuals based on information obtained at the level of the group. Often there may not be homogeneity of exposure of individuals in an area, although all individuals in an assigned exposure category will be assumed to be equally exposed (Greenland, 1992). This could lead to what is referred to as the 'ecological fallacy': an apparent association at the group level may not hold at the individual level. Where air pollution levels are fairly uniformly distributed in an area, and microvariations are of little significance, this type of problem is less likely to arise.

Other problems relate to the fact that information on potentially confounding factors is frequently absent, so that the relationship between exposure and outcome may be distorted. In addition, exposure and outcome data are usually not available for exactly corresponding areas. Thus, it may be difficult to convert existing health and environmental data into corresponding units of analysis. Frequently, proxy (substitute) measures of exposures and outcomes are used. Nevertheless, despite their limitations, they are relatively easy and quick to conduct using existing databases.

Studies that have relied on this type of design include cancer studies in which, for example, lung cancer rates in different parts of a region are analysed in relation to air pollution levels estimated on the basis of air monitoring data in the region, or in relation to types of industry in the region. They can often yield useful information and early clues, which can then be further pursued using different study designs.

Geographic Information Systems (GIS)

These can be used to organize, analyse and present data at the community level. They can range from very sophisticated and well developed systems that require substantial inputs in terms of data and equipment, to very simple systems that can be run on microcomputers and economical, user-friendly software (Scholten and de Lepper, 1991). Whilst a large scale GIS is not a rapid assessment method in itself, once the initial investment of setting up such a system has been made, information can be retrieved quickly. In addition, in a rapid assessment it is extremely useful to be able to draw on the facility of a GIS to present data in map form. Maps are easy to understand and use, which makes them attractive as communication tools (Anker, 1991).

The GIS can be very useful for providing a method of analysis that relates specifically to the geographical component of the data. At the simplest level, data about different spatial entities such as land use and air pollution can be combined by overlay analysis. At an intermediate level GIS may allow statistical calculations of the relationships between datasets to be computed. The most sophisticated analysis occurs when modelling is introduced. Atmospheric modelling techniques can be used to discover which areas might be affected by pollution resulting from an explosion at a particular hazardous installation, for example Chernobyl, given certain wind and weather conditions. It can also be used to assess the impact of locating a specific industrial development in different sites in a city or region.

The compilation of maps and atlases can show how patterns of spatial distribution of disease can be revealed. They can be useful for looking for clusters of diseases in relation to industries such as nuclear reprocessing facilities or hazardous waste incinerators. GIS has been used, for example, in looking at the relationship between perinatal mortality and radiation fallout from Chernobyl. It provides a method to perform various tasks more quickly and with less effort, and provides researchers with new, reliable, scientifically valid methods for handling spatial information (Scholten and de Lepper, 1991). Costs of hardware have declined substantially and a range of simple, introductory level systems now exist.

Time-series study

A variation on these designs is the time-series study, in which changes in health outcome in an area are looked at in relation to changing air pollution levels (Dockery and Pope, 1996). For example, daily hospital admissions or emergency room visits could be assessed in relation to daily air pollution levels (eg particulates), and acute effects such as asthma examined. As these studies are concerned with examining changes in air pollution levels and associated health effects, extraneous or confounding factors (eg smoking) are more effectively controlled because they would not be expected to vary in the same manner as the exposures under consideration. Whilst these studies are useful for studying the relationship between transient exposures and acute health effects, they are not, however, of use in studying chronic health effects. They can also be statistically and computationally demanding.

Such studies have been used to assess the relationship between daily mortality, air pollution and weather (Dockery and Pope, 1996; WHO, 1996), and were used to assess the impact of major air pollution episodes such as the London smog disasters in the 1950s. They also have application in studying the effects of the recent air pollution episodes in Asia and Latin America caused by forest fires.

Sentinel surveillance

Surveillance refers to the need for continual monitoring and observation of the distribution and trends of selected health outcomes and exposures, with a view to acting when certain limits are passed. It is needed to continually monitor change. This is particularly important during a period of rapid urbanization and industrial development, for example when there could be significant impacts on health arising from air pollution. Frequently, however, the data collected are not presented in a way that facilitates rapid action or which informs decision-making. On occasion too many data are collected, with a loss of quality and accuracy, or too few data are collected, or data are collected too infrequently, or at inappropriate sites, or in such a way that an analysis or action is not timely. Frequently, the best surveillance is found where the risk is smallest.

Because of the lack of resources and the burden of routine surveillance, sentinel surveillance sites can be identified in order to measure the health status of the population without studying the entire population, or the concept could be expanded to include a list of tracer health conditions that could trigger a study. This could be useful in emergency situations where time constraints are critical (Guha-Sapir, 1991) and early warning signs of impending disasters are needed, based on key indicators and sentinel surveillance systems.

RISK ASSESSMENT

Occasionally, there may be no health data and no possibility of obtaining such data; in this case a risk assessment may need to be conducted. Risk assessment has been widely used as a basis for setting standards, and has primarily involved three major categories of human health effects, namely carcinogenicity, developmental toxicity and neurotoxicity. The methodology, however, has broad relevance and applicability to other situations in which there is a lack of data on health effects in a particular setting.

Risk assessment has been defined by Griffith et al (1993) as 'the characterization of potential adverse health effects of human exposures to environmental hazards'. It involves the following steps, as first recommended by the US National Academy of Sciences (National Research Council, 1983):

1   hazard identification;
2   dose–response assessment;
3   exposure assessment; and
4   risk characterization.

Hazard identification is concerned with establishing whether an agent actually causes a specific effect. Dose–response assessment is concerned with establishing the relationship between the dose or exposure and the incidence of health effects in humans, whilst exposure assessment is concerned with identifying the exposures that are currently experienced or anticipated under different conditions. Risk characterization involves determining the estimated incidence of the adverse effect in a given population.

Hazard identification

Here one is concerned with establishing whether causal relationships exist between various exposures and health effects. As already discussed, this is a complex process. There are many factors that characterize the nature of the relationship between exposure to air pollution and health effects, which should be taken into account in trying to impute the nature of associations. On occasion there may be very little epidemiological information available, and therefore reliance must be placed on toxicological studies or on a combination of epidemiological and toxicological studies.

Dose–response

One is concerned here in establishing whether at increasing levels of exposure or dose there is a corresponding increase in the frequency or the severity of disease. This step involves the quantitative aspect of the assessment. For example, lung cancer incidence is known to rise in relation to cigarette smoking. Another example is lead exposure, where it may be possible to show a rise in the prevalence of raised blood lead levels with increasing levels of lead in petrol, or an increase in the incidence of neurobehavioural disorders in infants with increases in cord blood lead levels.

Information is usually obtained on the basis of the epidemiological literature, supported by animal toxicological and clinical data. Those scientific studies that are likely to show the best evidence of an effect would be selected for assessment. Whilst no single study is likely to be definitive on its own, the duplication of results across several studies and a range of exposures and health outcomes is strong evidence of a causal relationship (see earlier discussion on this aspect), and can be used for establishing the nature of the dose–response effect.

There is a wealth of scientific literature that can be consulted for this purpose, including the WHO air quality guidelines (WHO, 1987; WHO, 1999a) and various environmental health criteria documents on specific pollutants. Unfortunately, most of the data are derived from studies carried out in developed countries; nevertheless, there are now several studies from developing countries, which can also be consulted (see also accompanying chapters). Extreme caution needs to be exercized in extrapolating results from developed countries, as factors such as susceptibility of groups at risk, influencing factors such as diet and nutrition, and the role of background factors in the home, work and community environment are likely to differ significantly.

Exposure assessment

Here one is concerned with providing an estimate of human exposure levels from all potential sources for particular population groups under consideration in the assessment. Of critical importance is that major pollution sources in terms of population exposures are well identified and characterized in order that control strategies can be developed. One would need to provide an assessment of the size and composition of the population groups potentially exposed, and the types, magnitude, frequency and duration of exposure to the various agents of concern. All pathways of exposure would need to be assessed, for example not only the direct inhalation pathway, but also, in some cases, indirect pathways of air pollution exposure such as via food, water or the skin. This is one of the most challenging issues in air pollution epidemiology due to the complexities involved in estimating exposures, particularly personal exposures.

Risk characterization

This involves estimating the likely incidence of an adverse health effect resulting from exposure to a specific air pollutant. The information obtained on people's exposures can be used to determine how much of an agent will reach people, and the combination of this information with what is known of the dose–response relationship, based for example on scientific assessments and reviews, can be used to characterize people's risks. Essentially, in this step the information from hazard identification, dose–response relationships and exposure estimates is integrated to determine the probability of risk to humans.

COLLECTION OF INDIVIDUAL AND AGGREGATE LEVEL DATA

In all of the above assessments, data need to be collected on health outcomes and exposures, either at the individual or at the group level. If there is an interest in morbidity, in cases where formal disease registries exist, for example for cancer, these can be utilized. Other routine health surveillance and recording systems could also be used, for example hospital records (admission or discharge records), clinic or health service records, school and workplace records, or routine data on infectious diseases such as pneumonia. If there is an interest in mortality, most countries have routine data on causes of death, although cause-specific mortality may be subject to misclassification.

In situations where such data sources are limited, special surveys may be needed. The particular methods and techniques used to assess health effects would depend on the health effect of interest.

Focus group discussions and questionnaires

Questionnaires and focus group discussions may be used to obtain a quick impression of potential health effects (and exposures) in communities fairly rapidly. Data can be collected on an aggregate level in many ways, including using groups of experts, community leaders, individuals from the community, in-depth interviews with selected individuals, etc. Focus group interviews can be used to obtain important in-depth qualitative data, for example to examine local perceptions. Simple self-administered questionnaires can also be distributed, which can form the basis for more substantial quantitative studies. They can be very useful for investigating people's knowledge, attitudes and behaviour, and it can be important to conduct them prior to designing interventions.

In addition, they can be useful for pinpointing at-risk areas or populations, or issues in need of further study. Often they are used as a complement to a quantitative study. They are useful also in providing background information and to generate hypotheses for field testing, but would rarely be used as a stand-alone method (Khan et al, 1991).

Questionnaires are also invaluable for obtaining information from key informants in the community (Lengeler et al, 1991), and can be a useful alternative to the direct interview approach. Self-reports of symptoms are often used as a health outcome in studies with uncertain exposures and few or no objectively measurable health effects. However, over-reporting of symptoms may occur in groups who are aware of their exposure to air pollution (Mendell, 1990). Examples of such situations include communities worried about toxic waste site exposures, or office workers concerned about indoor air pollution.

Exposure assessments

Multiple sources and pathways

There are normally multiple sources and pathways of exposure that would need to be assessed. For example, people could become exposed to lead in petrol via the air they breathe, the food they eat, or via soil and dust that may get ingested. Often one pathway contributes the major proportion of the pollutant. Should this critical pathway not be identified, the multiple pathways contributing to the total exposure must be carefully assessed. Adequate control measures can only be applied when the relative importance of the various routes of exposure has been established.

People may be exposed to various sources of the same agent in addition to the various pathways of uptake. For example, lead may be present in petrol, paint or drinking water. Often there may be multiple sources in differing environments that may contribute to the same health outcome, for example, in the domestic (home) environment, the local or community environment, the school or work environment, etc (von Schirnding et al, 1990). For young children and women, the indoor environment may be a particularly important source of exposure, especially in developing countries where exposures to biomass and coal may be significant (see Chapter 7); for adults, the workplace may be an important source of exposure. Thus, it is important to assess an individual's total exposure in the various environments in which exposure may take place, as well as to identify other substances that may modify its effects.

Variations in time and space

Exposures may also vary considerably in time and space. For example, for many pollutants there is a sharp decrease in concentration level as one moves away from a source. There may also be significant vertical variations in the concentration level of a pollutant. For example, air sampling points placed considerably above breathing level may be safe from vandalism but are inappropriate in population exposure studies.

Similarly, there may be temporal variations (seasonal, daily and diurnal) in the level of pollution. For example, pollutant levels may vary throughout the day with respect to particulate levels associated with biomass burning for cooking and heating. These may reach peak levels in the early morning and early evening when cooking activities take place.

There may also be long term variations in exposure over time, during which sources (and pathways) may have changed. In investigating acute effects (see earlier discussion on this aspect) the current exposure level may be adequate, but in studying chronic effects (after a long exposure period or latency period) past exposure concentration levels are important, as well as the duration of exposure.

Problems in relying on both historical and current environmental measurements may arise due to the fact that the measurement technology may have changed over time, with current technology increasingly able to measure at lower detection levels.

Techniques for assessing exposure to air pollutants

There are many ways, both directly and indirectly, of classifying a person's exposure: it could be on the basis of the nearest air pollution monitor, on a weighted average of all the monitors in an area, on some dispersion modelling scheme in which different areas are designated different values, on the basis of source emissions data, on the basis of personal exposure measures, or merely on the basis of a residential classification scheme. It can be done at the aggregate level or at the individual level.

The specifics of an exposure assessment will depend on its purpose, ie the nature of the information required. The quantity and quality of data required will depend on the context for which they are needed. Whilst here the main concern is in obtaining an overall assessment of exposure as rapidly as possible, nevertheless the way in which air pollutants are monitored will always be a critical aspect (UNEP, 1994). A great deal of monitoring information is of limited use due to the fact that it may not be relevant to where people are exposed, or pollutants may not be measured frequently enough.

There are several problems involved in relying on stationary environmental monitoring schemes. Pollutants are typically measured at only a limited number of sites, and often the schemes are designed to determine compliance with air quality standards and not to assess exposure. Thus, they may not provide estimates of average pollution levels to which people are typically exposed, but would be useful for other purposes, for example in assessing long term trends and emissions from point sources. Dispersion modelling can also be used to obtain more reliable estimates of air pollution exposures.

Personal sampling

Where microvariations in pollutant levels are considerable it may be more appropriate to use personal air samplers or filter badges rather than stationary air samplers. These have the advantage of being mobile and have the potential to measure an individual's total exposure. Examples of personal monitoring include diffusion tubes for passively sampling gases, or filters with battery-operated pumps for actively sampling aerosols.

If large populations are being monitored, however, such samplers may not be practicable and exposures might be better characterized at the group level using stationary samplers. They could be very useful, however, in small area studies or in studies of particular risk groups such as young children or workers. Radiation dosimeters are an example of this type of monitoring. In general, however, they tend to be relatively expensive and labour intensive, sometimes requiring fairly sophisticated analytical procedures and laboratory facilities as well as detailed information on time activity patterns (WHO, 1999b).

Proxy measures and source emissions inventories

Where no air pollution measurements exist proxies can be used, such as place of residence (for example, urban, suburban, inner city, industrial zone). Dispersion modelling can also be used, provided that there are relatively accurate inventories of emission sources. In Jakarta, for example, dispersion models that take into account local meteorological and topographical features have been used to determine ambient concentrations throughout the region, and individuals' assigned exposures based on their place of residence (WHO, 1996). Weighted exposures might also be assigned, based on residence and workplace for example.

Many methods for assessing sources of air pollution exist, for example, in calculating pollution and waste loads. While detailed and precise source emission inventories can be resource intensive, involving sophisticated monitoring and data processing systems, by using limited existing information it is possible to make fairly accurate emission inventories at fairly low cost (WHO, 1982).

The methods involve obtaining information on types and sizes of waste and pollution sources, as well as information on their location (for example, in relation to population centres); pollution and waste loads can then be calculated on the basis of pollution and waste factors for the various sources. Many factors need to be taken into account including, for example, the source type, age, technological sophistication, process or design particularities, source maintenance and operating practices, raw materials used and control systems employed, etc (WHO, 1993b).

Separate inventories could be made for areas with point sources and areas with mobile sources. Estimated emissions for stationary combustion sources, mobile combustion engine sources, industrial processes, waste disposal processes and so on could be tabulated, and contributions of sources to air pollution loads estimated, taking into account meteorological conditions and the locations of sources. This can be conducted fairly crudely, or it can involve very sophisticated source apportionment studies. Decisions need to be made in relation to whether data are required for individual sources or for groups of sources: in situations where there are a few large sources such as electric power plants, individual level data are probably required, whereas in situations where there are numerous small sources such as space heating furnaces, joint calculations will be necessary (WHO, 1993b).

Various tools for the rapid assessment of air pollutants have been developed (see also WHO's Air Management Information System (AMIS) and the Decision Support System for Industrial Pollution Control (DSS IPC)) and mostly include information on emission factors for various sources, models for pollution dispersion taking into account meteorological data (for example, wind speed and direction, temperature), and methods for estimating pollutant concentrations. Thus, the steps involved would include making an inventory of key air polluting activities, compiling an inventory of emissions of pollutants based on emission factors, and calculating ambient concentrations based on dispersion modelling, for example. Where direct emissions data are missing, various sources can be consulted on industrial emission factors, or on transport emission factors for example, which are based on data for various fuels and vehicles.

Biological markers of exposure

There is growing interest and increasing research into biological and biochemical markers of exposure (WHO, 1993c), which should improve the effectiveness of exposure assessments in the future. Concentrations of air pollutants in body fluids or excreta may be measured – for example, through the biological monitoring of blood, urine and hair. These can also be useful for estimating past exposure levels, for example measurement of lead levels in bones or hair. The advantage is that they provide integrated measures of exposures from all sources and pathways. Those most suitable would be chemical specific, detectable in trace quantities, available by non-invasive techniques (eg urine) and inexpensive to assay (WHO, 1999b). Sources of biological variability need to be taken into account in interpreting the data (age, sex, body size, fat distribution, lifestyle factors, other sources of exposure).

Summary

In summary, exposure information provides the critical link between sources of contaminants, their presence in the environment and their health impacts. Assessments can be direct or indirect, based on monitoring and interpolation of data from monitoring sites, source emissions inventories and dispersion modelling, or can even be based on questionnaire data at the individual level (see earlier discussion on this aspect) or on biological markers in individuals.

Ultimately, the exposure data must be summarized: the choice of an appropriate summary measure may be critical to the ultimate understanding of the exposure. In one instance average exposure level may be appropriate, while in another the use of peak values may be important. Cumulative exposures may be of significance in the assessment of, for example, radiation exposure where multiple exposures may be largely cumulative. Thus, one might choose the average, peak, percentile, frequency of exceedance of a specified level, or cumulative duration of exceedance.

CONCLUSIONS

The relationship between air pollution and health is complex. A wide variety of factors influence the association between exposures and health effects in human populations in any one setting or at-risk group. Decision-makers are frequently faced with the need to make rapid appraisals of situations, often based on sparse data on exposure, health effects or their associations.

This chapter has discussed the need for rapid appraisals, the circumstances in which they may be necessary, their distinguishing characteristics, and some of the assessment methods that can be used, relying on information either at the level of the individual or at the group level. The specifics of the situation will determine the method(s) to be used.

Ultimately, there is no replacement for well designed epidemiological or risk assessment studies. Rapid appraisals should thus never be considered in isolation, but should rather be seen as part of an overall air pollution health effects assessment programme that is updated and developed over time.

REFERENCES

Anker, M (1991) 'Epidemiological and statistical methods for rapid health assessment' in *World Health Statistics Quarterly*, vol 44, no 3

Armstrong, J and Campbell, H (1991) 'Indoor air pollution exposure and lower respiratory infections in young Gambian children' in *International Journal of Epidemiology*, vol 20, no 2

Baltazar, J (1991) 'The potential of the case control method for rapid epidemiological assessment' in *World Health Statistics Quarterly*, vol 44, no 3

Bradford Hill, A (1965) 'The environment and disease: association or causation?' in *Proceedings of the Royal Society of Medicine*, vol 58

Dockery, D and Pope, A (1996) 'Epidemiology of acute health effects: summary of time-series studies' in R Wilson and J Spengler (eds) *Particles in Our Air: Concentration and Health Effects*, Harvard University Press, Geneva

Goldsmith, J (1986) *Epidemiological Investigation of Community Environmental Health Problems*, CRC Press Inc, Boca Raton

Goldsmith, J (1988) 'Improving the prospects for environmental epidemiology' in *Archives of Environmental Health*, vol 43, no 2

Greenland, S (1992) 'Divergent biases in ecologic and individual-level studies' in *Statistics in Medicine*, vol 11

Griffith, J, Aldrich, T and Drane, W (1993) 'Risk assessment' in T Aldrich and J Griffith (eds) *Environmental Epidemiology and Risk Assessment*, Van Nostrand Reinhold, New York

Guha-Sapir, D (1991) 'Rapid assessment of health needs in mass emergencies: review of current concepts and methods' in *World Health Statistics Quarterly*, vol 44, no 3

Khan, M, Anker, M, Patel, B, Barge, S, Sadhwani, H and Kohle, R (1991) 'The use of focus groups in social and behavioural research: some methodological issues' in *World Health Statistics Quarterly*, vol 44, no 3

Lengeler, C, Mshinda, H, de Savigny, D, Kilima, P, Morona, D and Tanner, M (1991) 'The value of questionnaires aimed at key informants, and distributed through an existing administrative system, for rapid and cost-effective health assessment' in *World Health Statistics Quarterly*, vol 44, no 3

Lilienfeld, A and Lilienfeld, D (1980) *Foundations of Epidemiology*, Oxford University Press, Oxford

Mausner, J and Kramer, S (1985) *Epidemiology: An Introductory Text*, W B Saunders and Co, Philadelphia

Mendell, M (1990) *Data in Setting with Likely Over-reporting Due to Environmental Worry*, 2nd Annual Meeting of the International Society for Environmental Epidemiology, US, 12–15 August

National Research Council (1983) *Risk Assessment in the National Government: Managing the Process*, National Academy Press, Washington, DC

Pope, A and Dockery, D (1996) 'Epidemiology of chronic health effects: cross-sectional studies' in R Wilson and J Spengler (eds) *Particles in Our Air: Concentration and Health Effects*, Harvard University Press, Cambridge, MA

Robin, L, Less, P, Winget, M, Steinhoff, M, Moulton, L, Santosham, M and Correa, A (1996) 'Wood-burning stoves and lower respiratory illnesses in Navajo children' in *Paediatric Infectious Disease Journal*, vol 15, no 10

Rothman, K (1986) *Modern Epidemiology*, Little, Brown and Co, New York

Scholten, H and de Lepper, M (1991) 'The benefits of the application of geographical information systems in public and environmental health' in *World Health Statistics Quarterly*, vol 44, no 3

UNEP/WHO (1994) *GEMS/AIR Methodology Review Handbook Series*, volumes 1, 2 and 3, United nations Environment Programme, Nairobi

von Schirnding, Y (1990) 'Methodological issues in air pollution epidemiology', Proceedings of the 1st IUAPPA Regional Conference on Air Pollution, South Africa, 24–26 October

von Schirnding, Y (1997) 'Environmental epidemiology' in J Katzenellenbogen et al (eds) *Epidemiology: A Manual for South Africa*, Oxford University Press, Cape Town

von Schirnding, Y, Bradshaw, D, Fuggle, R and Stokol, M (1990) 'Blood lead levels in inner-city South African children' in *Environmental Health Perspectives*, vol 94, pp125–130

WHO (1982) 'Rapid assessment of sources of air, water and land pollution' in *WHO Offset Publication*, no 62

WHO (1983) 'Guidelines on studies in environmental epidemiology' in *Environmental Health Criteria*, vol 27

WHO (1987) 'Air quality guidelines for Europe' in *European Series*, vol 23

WHO (1993a) *Basic Epidemiology*, WHO, Geneva

WHO (1993b) *Assessment of Sources of Air, Water and Land Pollution*, WHO/PEP/GETNET/93.1-A.P, WHO, Geneva

WHO (1993c) *Biomarkers and Risk Assessment: Concepts and Principles*, EHC 155, WHO, Geneva

WHO (1996) *A Methodology for Estimating Air Pollution Health Effects*, WHO, Geneva

WHO (1998) *Methods for Health Impact Assessment in Environmental and Occupational Health*, WHO, Geneva

WHO (1999a) *(Revised) Air Quality Guidelines for Europe* (second edition), WHO, Copenhagen

WHO (1999b) *Human Exposure Assessment*, WHO, Geneva

6

A Systematic Approach to Air Quality Management: Examples from the URBAIR Cities

Steinar Larssen, Huib Jansen, Xander A Olsthoorn, Jitendra J Shah, Knut Aarhus and Fan Changzhong

ABSTRACT

Urban air quality management in megacities is a complex task, which to be effective requires a sound understanding of the causes and effects of air pollution and its various components. As indicated in Chapter 4, the factual basis should ideally include data on emissions, actual air quality, source–exposure–effects relationships and assessment of damage and its costs. Such information can be used to construct a coherent action plan, with control measures prioritized according to cost-effectiveness or cost–benefit ratios. With continued monitoring it is possible to assess the results of the measures selected and implemented. The URBAIR project, financed through the World Bank, employed an air quality management system approach to help develop action plans in four large cities in Asia (Jakarta, Kathmandu, Manila and Mumbai). This chapter draws on the experience of the URBAIR project and more recent work in Guangzhou in China, and describes the procedures involved and the policy recommendations.

URBAN AIR QUALITY MANAGEMENT AND THE URBAIR PROJECT

The Urban Air Quality Management Strategy (URBAIR) project developed a systematic approach for the design and implementation of policies, monitoring systems and management mechanisms to restore ambient air quality in metropolitan areas. This approach has been applied and tested in Jakarta,

Mumbai and Metro Manila. These experiences can provide lessons for other metropolitan authorities.

The URBAIR project adopted an air quality management strategy (AQMS) involving the following steps:

- air quality assessment;
- environment and health damage assessment;
- abatement options assessment;
- cost–benefit analysis (CBA) or cost-effectiveness analysis;
- abatement measures selection (action plan); and
- design of optimum control strategy.

The main elements of the approach can be grouped as follows:

Assessment: Air quality assessment, environmental damage assessment and abatement options assessment provide input to the cost analysis, which is also based on established air quality objectives (eg air quality standards) and economic objectives (eg reduction of damage costs). The analysis leads to an action plan containing abatement and control measures for implementation in the short, medium and long term. The goal of this analysis is an optimum control strategy.

The AQMS depends on the following set of technical and analytical tasks, which can be undertaken by the relevant air quality authorities:

- creating an inventory of polluting activities and emissions;
- monitoring air pollution and dispersion parameters;
- calculating air pollution concentrations with dispersion models;
- assessing exposure and damage;
- estimating the effect of abatement and control measures; and
- establishing and improving air pollution regulations and policy measures.

These activities, and the institutions necessary to carry them out, constitute the prerequisites for establishing the AQMS.

Action plans and implementation: Categories of 'actions' include the following:

- technical abatement measures;
- improvements of the factual database (eg emission inventory, monitoring, etc);
- institutional strengthening;
- implementing an investment plan; and
- awareness-raising and environmental education.

Monitoring: A third essential component of AQMS is continued monitoring or surveillance. Monitoring is essential to assessing the effectiveness of air pollution control actions. The goal of an Air Quality Information System

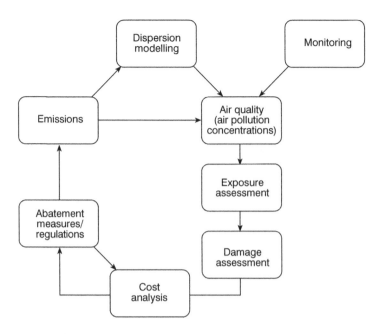

Figure 6.1 *The system for developing an Air Quality Management Strategy (AQMS) based upon assessment of effects and costs*

(AQIS) is, through thorough monitoring, to keep authorities, major polluters and the public informed about the short and long term changes in air quality, thereby helping to raise awareness; and to assess the results of abatement measures, thereby providing feedback to the abatement strategy.

Figure 6.1 describes how the necessary activities of an AQMS system should be linked together in an integrated system that enables abatement measures to be prioritized on the basis of cost-efficiency or CBA.

The URBAIR guidebook (Shah, Nagpal and Brandon, 1997) gives a detailed description of the methodologies that can be used to carry out these activities. Where a methodology is described in this chapter without a reference, please refer to the URBAIR guidebook.

In the URBAIR project, which was carried out from 1993 to 1996, action plans for improved air quality were developed for four Asian cities: Jakarta, Kathmandu, Manila and Mumbai (Shah and Nagpal 1997a, 1997b, 1997c, 1997d). In the following, the process of developing an AQMS is described briefly, using examples from the four URBAIR cities.

Following the completion of the URBAIR project, the URBAIR AQMS concept has been used to develop cost-effective action plans against air pollution in some cities in China, the city of Guangzhou in Guangdong province being the primary example (Larssen, 2000). Here the quantitative calculations of cost-effectiveness of various control options were carried further than for the URBAIR cities and an action plan with prioritized control options was constructed. This paper concludes by using the Guangzhou action plan as an example of the fuller use of the URBAIR AQMS concept.

PHYSICAL ASSESSMENT

Assessment of present air quality and choice of air quality indicators

The starting point for the air quality improvement study is to assess present air quality. If data of adequate quality are not available, a monitoring programme must be established (see for example Shah, Nagpal and Brandon, 1997; Larssen, 1998). It should be emphasized that it is very important that the data are of known and acceptable quality (Larssen and Helmis, 1998). The choice of pollutants to be used as indicators of the air quality situation depends upon the composition and extent of sources in the city. Experience with air quality assessment in Asian cities indicates that, in general, SO_2, NO_x, NO_2, ozone and particulate matter (PM) are the urban pollutants responsible for most of the potential damage (WHO, 1992). Air quality guidelines are available for these compounds, and much effort has been put into developing dose–response relationships for damage assessment. Another pollutant given increasing attention is benzene.

For the URBAIR cities, there were data available from various measurement campaigns, and monitoring systems were in routine operation in all of the cities except Kathmandu. The URBAIR project concentrated on the assessment of damage to health, and on the compounds SO_2, NO_x, NO_2 and PM.

The air quality assessment indicated that the PM problem was the most important in all cities. Table 6.1 gives a brief overview of the total suspended particles (TSP) concentrations measured in each city. In Mumbai, Manila and Jakarta, TSP measurements are made typically every sixth day at a number of stations, while in Kathmandu the data are from a three-month measurement campaign at several stations in 1993.

For assessment of health effects, PM_{10} is a more appropriate measure of suspended particles than TSP. PM_{10} measurements were scarce in these cities. Using commonly applied rules of thumb involving ratios of PM_{10} to TSP of between 0.5 and 0.6, it was found that annual PM_{10} concentrations in the cities would be up to 80–140 micrograms per cubic metre ($\mu g/m^3$). Maximum 24-hour PM_{10} concentrations would run as high as about $400\mu g/m^3$.

As indicated in Chapter 4, recent evidence indicates that there may be no concentration level below which there are no health effects of PM_{10} (WHO, 1994, 1996). Nevertheless, the European Union (EU) has target values (EU, 1998). The target for annual average of PM_{10} is 30–40$\mu g/m^3$ (to be reached in 2005 and 2010 respectively), while the 24-hour target is 50$\mu g/m^3$, which can be exceeded a certain number of times per year. The 24-hour target value corresponds to a maximum 24-hour value of some 80–100$\mu g/m^3$. The US Environmental Protection Agency (EPA) has proposed similar standards (US EPA, 1997).

The prevailing PM guideline and target values indicated that PM was the most serious ambient air pollution problem in these cities, and this was used as an indicator for assessing the potential health damage caused by air pollution.

Table 6.1 *Summary of measured TSP concentrations ($\mu g/m^3$) in four URBAIR cities*

	Mumbai 1992–1993	Manila 1990–1992	Jakarta 1991	Kathmandu 1993
Annual average all stations	223 (118–265)	174 (114–255)	291 (159–648)	253 (87–430)
24-hour average maximum at any station	–	823	840	867
Range of maximum at each station	–	247–823	540–840	102–867

Emissions to air

It is important to put sufficient resources into the establishment of emission inventories in cities. This is one of the main pillars of a thorough air quality assessment. For the four URBAIR cities, it turned out that the inventory of vehicle exhaust emissions and the contributions from various vehicle categories could be fairly complete because all the cities had reasonable data about vehicle fleets and fuel consumption. In addition, some traffic data were available from the main road networks. This is likely to be the situation in a number of cities. A first estimate of emission factors can be selected from the literature (eg Faiz et al, 1996; Shah and Nagpal 1997a), and the same factors were used in all the URBAIR cities. The basis for calculating emissions from industry is less likely to be complete. Even if industrial fuel combustion emissions can be reasonably well estimated, the spatial distribution is likely to be difficult to establish due to a lack of data. Moreover, process emissions are difficult to estimate with reasonable accuracy in many cities. In the URBAIR study, only in Kathmandu valley, where the main process industry is brick production, could these emissions be estimated with any completeness and accuracy.

Figure 6.2 shows the relative contributions to PM emissions from road vehicles, other fuel combustion and refuse burning in the URBAIR cities. The total of PM emissions from these sources, which were estimated as tons per year per million inhabitants, is considerably different between the cities, being highest in Manila and lowest in Mumbai. This may, to some extent, reflect the different levels of completeness and quality in the emission data given and collected for each city. The need for quality assurance in emissions inventories should be acknowledged. In the URBAIR study this could be accomplished only incompletely.

The total *road traffic* (including the vehicle-induced resuspension from roads) accounts for 45–60 per cent of the emissions from the mentioned sources in Mumbai, Manila and Jakarta, and only 35 per cent in Kathmandu. There are marked differences in the contribution from *industrial fuel*: this is considerable in Manila, at 39 per cent, because industry uses large amounts of heavy fuel oil; in the other cities, industrial fossil fuel contributes only about 10 per cent. Regarding *domestic fuel*, wood contributes significantly in Kathmandu and to some extent in Mumbai (for cremation). *Domestic refuse* emissions are based on

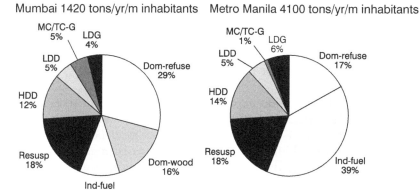

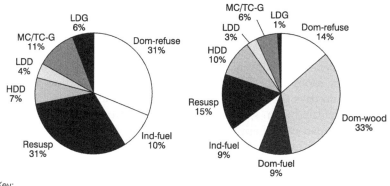

Key:
LDG = light duty vehicles, gasoline
LDD = light duty vehicles, diesel
HDD = heavy duty vehicles, diesel
MC/TC-G = motorcycles/tri-cycles, gasoline

Ind-fuel = industrial fossil fuel combination
Dom-wood = domestic wood combination
Dom-refuse = domestic refuse burning
Resusp = resuspension

Note: tons/yr/m inhabitants = tons per year per million inhabitants.

Figure 6.2 *Emission contributions to PM from various combustion source categories, plus road dust resuspension (RESUSP), in four URBAIR cities*

rather rough estimates, varying slightly between the cities. The source is estimated to contribute significantly.

The emissions from *industrial processes* must be added to the numbers in Figure 6.2. In Kathmandu, the brick industry adds emissions amounting to about 80 per cent of the emissions included in Figure 6.2.

Population exposure and assessment of health damage and its costs

The emissions should be distributed spatially according to the locations of the road network and other sources, and the population distribution. This, together with meteorological/dispersion parameter data, is then used as inputs to dispersion models that calculate the spatial distribution of concentrations and population exposure.

In the URBAIR study, a climatological, gaussian multisource model was used to calculate annual average concentrations in kilometre-squared grids over the cities. It is also possible to use more advanced dispersion models, which are increasingly available.

Using calculated population exposure distributions and dose–response relationships, the damage to the health of the population and its costs can be estimated. Many of the costs stem from the increased incidence of pollution-related illness and reduced life expectancy. The former is valued in terms of medical care costs and lost daily wages, as well as expenses undertaken to prevent illness. The latter is more difficult to evaluate in economic terms. The cost of increased mortality is based on value of a statistical life (VSL) estimates, either the willingness to pay (WTP) method or the human capital approach (see Shah, Nagpal and Brandon, 1997).

In the URBAIR study, the dose–response relationships developed by Ostro (1992, 1994) were used. For mortality and various morbidity indicators related to PM_{10} exposure, estimates of the extent of health damage were made. The morbidity indicators considered were chronic bronchitis, restricted activity days (RADs), emergency room visits (ERVs), bronchitis in children, asthma attacks, respiratory symptom days (RSDs) and respiratory hospital admissions (RHAs). The costs were calculated from specific costs per case of mortality (premature death) using the human capital approach and the morbidity indicators. These specific costs were estimated for each city based upon input from local consultants. The mortality cost is calculated as the discounted value of expected (average) future income at the average age of the population.

Table 6.2 shows the calculated health impact from PM_{10} in the cities in terms of the number of cases per million inhabitants, and the total annual costs associated with the entire impact in each city. The differences reflect the size of the population affected, the air pollution levels and the cost-per-case estimate made in each city, as well as the rate of the local currency relative to the US dollar. The estimated costs of the health effects were substantial: more than US$100 million per year in Mumbai, Manila and Jakarta.

In all cities, the costs related to sickness were higher than those estimated for mortality. This relation depends on the method used to value the costs of lives lost. For example, much higher mortality costs than those presented would result if US WTP estimates were applied.

COST–BENEFIT ANALYSIS OF SELECTED MEASURES

After having established an estimate of the damage associated with the present pollution level in a city, a comparison of the economic costs and benefits associated with the introduction of selected pollution control measures can be carried out:

Table 6.2 *Estimated annual health impacts and their costs related to PM$_{10}$ pollution in the four URBAIR cities*

	Mumbai 1991	Metro Manila 1992	Jakarta 1990	Kathmandu Valley 1993
Exposure (% of population)*				
TSP>90µg/m^3	97%	67%	>99%	50%
TSP>180µg/m^3	5%	15%	~50%	3–4%
Health impact from PM$_{10}$ (cases per 10^6 inhabitants)				
mortality	279	155	459	79
morbidity				
chronic bronchitis	2000	1430	n/c	477
RADs (10^3)	1870	1310	3265	448
ERVs	7600	5360	13,370	1835
bronchitis in children	19,000	13,330	33,000	4575
asthma attacks	74,100	51,900	130,000	17,800
RSDs (10^3)	6000	4170	10,410	1430
respiratory hospital admissions	400	238	714	93
Monetary value of health impact:	*US$ millions*	*US$ millions*	*US$ millions*	*US$ millions*
total city mortality**	22.7	18.8	49.7	0.57
morbidity***				
RADs	17.2	67.7	69.4	0.53
asthma attacks	24.3	19.8	6.9	0.23
RSDs	39.0	59.1	1.6	1.51

Notes: * = exposure at residences. The high end of the population exposure, near roads and other sources, and its effects is not included.
** = the human capital approach was employed to estimate the VSL.
*** = selected morbidity indicators which represent the largest health costs (monetary value).
n/c = not calculated.

- select feasible measures which, evaluated from the emissions inventory and other information, have the potential to significantly reduce the pollution level, the population exposure and thus the damage;
- estimate the costs related to the implementation of the measures, implemented to the extent feasible and necessary; and
- estimate the reduction in the damage (the benefit in monetary terms) associated with the implementation of the measures by running the health damage calculations (emissions, dispersion, exposure) with the reduced emissions implemented.

For the principles of CBA, the reader is referred to the URBAIR guidebook (Shah, Nagpal and Brandon, 1997) and to Mishan (1988).

This analysis was carried out for each of the URBAIR cities. The results of the CBA of selected measures in Manila are shown in Table 6.3. Table 6.4 summarizes the CBA results for some of the measures in Mumbai, Manila and Jakarta. For Kathmandu, a CBA in monetary terms was not carried out.

Both costs and benefits of the selected measures vary between the cities (see the following section). However, for a number of the abatement measures in every city the benefits exceed the costs, in some cases substantially.

Action Plans

The development of an action plan for air pollution abatement involves several steps:

The first step is to identify the pollution abatement measures that are available, given the location and source composition of the city. This list of measures should be established early in a study, when an overview of sources and emissions has been made. In the URBAIR study, these abatement measures were sorted into five categories:

1   improved fuel quality;
2   technology improvement;
3   fuel switching;
4   traffic management; and
5   transport demand management.

The second step is to analyse each measure in terms of its costs, effectiveness (potential benefits), feasibility and any other factors of concern. The analysis is done according to the steps laid out in the previous section. In practice, only selected measures with a large potential and reasonable costs need to be analysed, at least in the first round.

In the URBAIR study, each city built its action plan in a slightly different way, but for each measure the following characteristics were described:

- what (description);
- how (policy instruments to instigate and implement the measure);
- when I (when actions should be implemented);
- when II (when results can be expected);
- who (institutions/organizations responsible or affected);
- effects (reduced emissions/exposure/damage costs);
- cost (cost of measure);
- feasibility (of the measure); and
- other (significant factors).

In addition to the measures that relate directly to reduced pollution, the action plan should also address the need to improve the basis for the air quality improvement strategy: improving the database (monitoring, emission inventory, modelling, etc) and the regulatory and institutional basis for establishing an operational air quality management system in the city.

The third step is to make a list of the selected measures prioritized according to their cost-effectiveness or cost–benefit ratio, their feasibility and the availability of policy instruments to facilitate their implementation. This list of measures, accompanied by an investment plan, forms the basis for the action plan. Listing the measures in order of priority indicates how many of them need to be implemented in order to reach the air quality target. Figure 6.3 gives a visualization of how to rank measures according to their cost-effectiveness (and their feasibility), ie the cost per ton of reduced emissions versus the total potential for population exposure reduction. It also indicates that some measures may give a net saving as well as reducing pollution (eg, if the measure saves fuel). The 'first' measures give significant effects at relatively low cost, and then costs increase and effects decrease as less efficient measures are chosen.

In the URBAIR cities the analysis was carried as far as is shown in Table 6.4, where the costs and benefits of selected, feasible measures are compared. The list reflects the importance of the pollution associated with road traffic in these cities (Mumbai, Manila and Jakarta). In Kathmandu, industrial brick production was of equal importance to road traffic.

Substantial benefits, larger than the estimated costs, were found for the following measures: unleaded gasoline, low-smoke lubrication oil (for two-stroke motorcycles), inspection/maintenance of vehicles (although considered more costly in Jakarta) and the control of gross polluters (eg vehicles with visible exhaust). Substantial benefits were also found for the following measures, but here the costs were estimated to be higher than the benefits: clean vehicle standards (state of the art) and cleaner fuel oils.

One potentially important measure is improved diesel quality. The costs are estimated to be much higher than the benefits in Mumbai, roughly the same as the benefits in Manila and probably less than the benefits in Jakarta. These differences probably reflect the different availability and pricing policies of fuels in the countries.

POLICY INSTRUMENTS AND PLANS FOR AIR QUALITY IMPROVEMENT IN URBAIR CITIES

The implementation of plans and strategies for air quality improvements is conventionally done through the use of policy instruments by ministries, regulatory agencies, law enforcers and other institutions. Indeed, some of these institutions may well be the same as those that must be in place to carry out the AQMS analysis described here, which ideally is the basis for the plans and strategies. Thus the existence of relevant institutions and an organizational institutional structure is part of the basis for AQMS work.

Table 6.3 *CBA of selected abatement measures in Manila, 1992 (annual costs)*

Abatement measure	Benefits		Cost of measure	Time frame	
	Avoided emissions,* tons PM$_{10}$ per year	Avoided health damage		Introduction of measure**	Effect of measure
Vehicles: addressing gross polluters					
Effective campaign against smoke-belching	2000	US$16–20 million, 158 deaths, 4 million RSDs	US$0.08 million	Immediate	Short term
Improving diesel quality	1200	US$10–12 million, 94 deaths, 2.5 million RSDs	US$10 million	Immediate	2–5 years
Inspection/ maintenance	4000	US$30–40 million, 316 deaths, 8 million RSDs	US$5.5 million	Immediate	2–5 years
Fuel switching: diesel to gasoline in vehicles	2000	US$59–73 million, 600 deaths, 15 million RSDs	Immediate		5–10 years
Clean vehicle standards (cars/vans)	7000	US$94–116 million, 895 deaths, 24 million RSDs	US$5–20 million	Immediate	5–10 years
Fuel combustion: cleaner fuel oil	5000	US$10–20 million, 100 deaths, 2.5 million RSDs	US$10–20 million	Immediate	1–2 years
Power plants: clean fuel	500	Small	US$10 million	Immediate	1–2 years

Notes: * = The various abatement measures are not necessarily independent of each other. Thus, the 'avoided emissions' stated in this table for each measure separately may not simply be added together to obtain an estimate of the total effect of packages of measures.
** = Time frame for starting the work necessary to introduce measure.

Institutions on different government levels: Different levels of government – national, regional and local – have different roles and responsibilities in the environmental sphere. Air quality standards or guidelines are usually set at the national level, although local government may have the legal right to impose stricter regulations. National governments usually assume the responsibility for scientific research and environmental education, while local governments develop and enforce regulations and policy measures to control local pollution levels.

Table 6.4 *Summary of CBA results, three URBAIR cities*

Abatement measure	Mumbai (1991) Benefits US$ millions	Costs	Manila (1992) Benefits US$ millions	Costs	Jakarta (1990) Benefits US$ millions	Costs
Unleaded gasoline	NQ	NQ	NQ	NQ	146	24
Low-smoke lubrication oil for 2-stroke motorcycles	4.9	1.0	n/a	16	1–5	
Inspection/ maintenance, vehicles	8.2	4.9–9.8	30–40	5.5	15	33
Control gross polluters	4.1	NQ (small)	16–20	0.01	12	Low
Clean vehicle standards: cars/vans	4.1	24.6	94—116	5–20	33	41
Motorcycles	7.8	19.7	n/a		NQ	NQ
Improved diesel quality	2.6	9.8	10—12	10	2.9	Low
50% compressed natural gas	2.5	NQ	NQ	NQ	6.7	NQ
Cleaner fuel oil	1.6	14.8	10—20	10–20	NQ	NQ

Note: NQ = not quantified.

In the context of an AQMS, local authorities have the most significant responsibilities. These include the following:

- developing and running the monitoring programme;
- assessing the air quality;
- determining the impacts of air pollution;
- setting goals for the quality of air; and
- developing future scenarios and action plans to achieve those goals.

National or state authorities may assume the responsibility for mandating controls, such as regulating fuel quality, setting emissions standards and providing financial resources or incentives for the private sector to reduce emissions.

Institutional arrangements, laws and regulations are important parts of an AQMS. Some impediments to successful air quality management in low and middle income cities are weak institutions that lack technical skills and political authority, enforcement agencies that often lack both the necessary information and the means to implement policy, and unclear legal and administrative procedures. Countries have their own political and administrative hierarchies and technical expertise that affect institutions, laws and regulations related to air pollution control.

Laws and regulations on air quality are generally in place in three of the URBAIR cities: Mumbai, Metro Manila and Jakarta. In Kathmandu, the

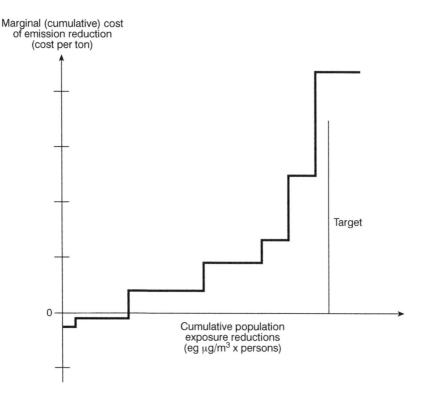

Figure 6.3 *Visualization of ranking of measures to reduce population exposure and thus health damage*

regulatory framework for controlling air pollution was still in an early phase. National clean air acts had been adopted. Standards for air quality and emissions and specifications of maximum amounts of pollutants in fuel (eg sulphur and lead) were also typically in place, as well as procedures of environmental impact assessment (EIA) for new establishments.

The analysis of institutions involved in air quality control and management in the four URBAIR cities revealed that national, regional (provincial) and local institutions were involved in all cities, to different degrees and with different tasks and divisions of responsibilities. The importance of clarity in the organizational structures and the division and description of responsibilities and lines of command must be stressed.

Various available *policy instruments* are described in the URBAIR guidebook (Shah, Nagpal and Brandon, 1997). It is important that the selected instruments do not have significant negative side effects within the environmental sphere or elsewhere. Social conditions and characteristics particular to a society must also be kept in mind. Within the local context, one can try to find the most effective or efficient instruments. An instrument that maximizes the effect (given a certain budget) or minimizes costs (given a certain environmental objective) should be chosen.

Policy instruments may be grouped into *direct regulation* (eg guidelines and standards for emission and air quality, enforcement of compliance, spatial planning and zoning and traffic regulations), *economic instruments* (eg emissions charges, taxes or subsidies, emissions trading) and instruments related to *communication and awareness-building*. Effective dissemination of information about pollution levels, contributions and effects is important in creating a sense of responsibility for environmental quality and the results of individual actions and practices. This is relevant for industry, product designers and other private sector actors, as well as individual citizens.

Clean air policy programmes: Two of the four URBAIR cities, Metro Manila and Jakarta, formulated policy programmes during the early 1990s for air quality improvement. OPLAN Clean Air Metro Manila was a five-year programme, begun in January 1993 and culminating in a Clean Air 2000 Action Plan. The results from the URBAIR project for Manila fed into this process.

The national Blue Sky Programme (*Langit Biru*) of Indonesia was launched in 1991 with control plans for selected stationary source categories and motor vehicles, including the control of black smoke and the introduction of unleaded gasoline. The URBAIR analysis for Jakarta provided an impetus to increase the efforts in this programme. The national plan was paralleled by Jakarta's Clean Air Programme (*Prodasih*).

EXAMPLE: THE GUANGZHOU ACTION PLAN FOR IMPROVED AIR QUALITY

The Guangzhou project

The Guangzhou action plan was developed under the Air Quality Management and Planning System for Guangzhou project carried out during the period 1996–2000, and financed by the Norwegian Department of Foreign Aid and Development (NORAD) (Larssen, 2000). The work carried out in this project by four Guangzhou and four Norwegian partner institutions[1] followed closely the URBAIR concept as outlined at the beginning of this chapter and in Figure 6.1.

The work concentrated on SO_2, NO_x and total suspended particulates (TSP). SO_2 and TSP in particular constitute significant air pollution problems in the city of Guangzhou, which has about 6 million inhabitants. The main sources of these problems are the use of coal in power plants and industrial boilers, and more diversified coal use by smaller enterprises (eg restaurants, small industries) as well as for domestic purposes. The rapidly increasing road traffic is also an important NO_x source.

Action plans were considered for both the short term (2001) and longer term (2010). So far the short term action plan is the one that has been most thoroughly analysed, and it is shown here as an example. Only control options that were feasible for implementation in the short term were considered for the 2001 action plan.

Table 6.5 *Abatement costs and emissions reduction potentials of various SO$_2$ control options*

Option	Cost per ton removed (Chinese yen, RMB)	Emissions reduction potential (tons per year)
Cogeneration of 9 main industrial sources	2550	12,000 (+16,500 tons particles)
SI in power plants and large industrial boilers	2250	55,000
Shut down 18 power plants, 200 megawatts (MW) or less	0*	25,000 tons (+ 7000 tons NO$_x$ + 27,000 tons particles)**
Shut down 13 power plants, 150MW or less	0*	16,500 tons SO$_2$ (+ 3300 tons NO$_x$ + 25,000 tons particles)**
All large point sources use low sulphur coal (shift from 0.75% sulphur to 0.5% sulphur)	4500	25,000 (maximum 33% of bituminous part of large point source total emissions)
All large point sources shift from bituminous (0.75% sulphur) to anthracite (0.5% sulphur)	4900	4500 tons (maximum 33% of anthracite part of large point source total emissions)
Wet FGD on 17 largest point sources	4500	50,000 tons
Fuel switch: taxis	17,000	675 tons (15,000 taxis) + 540 tons TSP
Fuel switch: 1000 buses	45,000	140 tons (1000 buses) + 110 tons particles
Fuel switch: third industry	540,000***	2000–3000 tons (2% of total emissions)
Moving 20 factories	72,400	500 tons (+ 130 tons NO$_x$ and 1150 tons particles)

Notes: * = lower range.
** = lower range; numbers assume that small plants' production is shifted entirely to big plants within study area.
*** = involves investment in gas pipe infrastructure.

The action plan for improving the SO$_2$ pollution situation

The following control options for reducing SO$_2$ emissions were analysed:

- sorbent injection (SI) – large point sources;
- shutting down small power plants;
- shifting to low sulphur (LS) coal;
- wet flue gas desulphurization (FGD) in the largest point sources;
- fuel switch (FS) for taxis from gasoline to liquefied petroleum gas (LPG);
- fuel switch for buses from diesel to LPG;
- cogeneration in eight industrial facilities;

Table 6.6 *SO$_2$ concentration reduction potential and costs for each control option*

Control option	Total costs	Concentration reduction potential (%)	Cost per % point reduced SO$_2$ concentration
Cogeneration in 9 industrial sources	−30 million	5.5%	−5.4 million
Shut down 13 small power plants	0*	8%	0*
SI in 60 large point sources	124 million	26%	4.8 million
Shift to 0.5% sulphur coal, 60 large point sources	112 million	12%	9.3 million
Wet FGD in 17 largest point sources	225 million	24%	9.4 million
Fuel switch: 15,000 taxis	11.5 million	0.6%	19 million
Moving 20 factories	36.2 million	1.4%	26 million
Fuel switch: 1000 buses	6.3 million	0.15%	42 million
Fuel switch: tertiary industry	1350 million	2.4%	560 million

Note: * = it is assumed here that the old plants are fully depreciated, and since their power production is taken over by larger plants with available extra capacity, the net cost to society is negligible. If it is assumed that these plants are operable for another five years, the estimated cost to society of shutting them down is some RMB4000 per tonne of SO$_2$ removed.

- fuel switch in tertiary industry; and
- moving 20 factories.

Each of these options was analysed in terms of its:

- cost (per ton removed emissions);
- emissions reduction potential (total tons removed on an annual basis); and
- concentration reduction potential (in terms of the percentage of the total SO$_2$ concentration in the most polluted area, the central urban area of the city).[2]

The results of the abatement costs and emission reduction potential are shown in Table 6.5.

Some of the options seem rather powerful in terms of reduced emissions. The estimated total SO$_2$ emissions in the city was approximately 145,000 tons per year (1995), while the most powerful SO$_2$ reduction options, SI in power plants and large industrial boilers (a total of 60 sources), could potentially reduce this by 55,000 tons per year.

In Table 6.6 the resulting SO$_2$ concentration reduction potential for central urban Guangzhou is given, as well as the cost-effectiveness of the control options in terms of cost per percentage point reduction in SO$_2$ concentration in the central parts of the city.[3] Here the cost-effectiveness is calculated for each

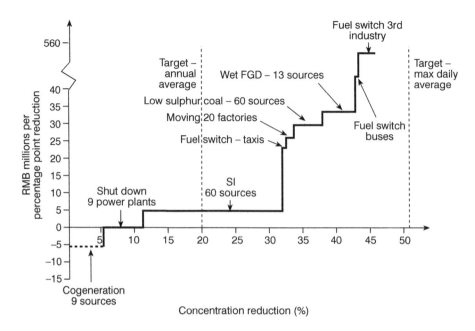

Figure 6.4 *Cost curve, SO₂ control options*

option separately. Cogeneration has a negative cost, representing a cost saving. SI is calculated as the most cost-effective of the other control options, while fuel switch for the tertiary industry (restaurants etc) has a high cost (because it involves large investments in gas piping systems etc) and small SO_2 concentration reduction potential.

When developing the action plan, the various control options must be considered together. Several options must usually be carried out to meet a set target for air quality, and they are often not mutually independent: the cost-effectiveness of a certain option is often dependent upon which control option have already been carried out.

The final result of the action plan development for SO_2 in Guangzhou is shown in Figure 6.4. The sequence of control options is given according to the cost-effectiveness of each option (in terms of concentration reduction), given that the 'previous' control options have already been carried out.

To meet the target for annual average concentrations of SO_2 (which is 60μg/m³), the SO_2 concentration in the central parts of Guangzhou should be reduced by about 20 per cent. This target is relatively easy to meet and requires cogeneration in nine specific large industrial boilers, shutting down nine small to medium size old power plants, and SI in the flue gases for a number of larger power plants and industrial boilers. The total annual costs for this package were calculated to be less than RMB70 million, which is quite moderate and certainly lower than the benefits involved in such a reduction.

The target for the maximum daily SO_2 concentration (which is 150μg/m³) is much more difficult to meet. If the first eight options are all implemented in

Table 6.7 *Total costs, concentration reduction potential and costs per percentage point of reduced concentrations for various control options*

Option	Total costs RMB	Concentration reduction potential	Cost per percentage point reduced NO_x concentration
Shut down 13 power plants, 150MW or less	0[*]	4%[*]	0[*]
LNB (and OFA) on 26 largest sources	40 million	11%	3.6 million
SNCR on 26 largest sources	66 million	12.2%	5.4 million
TWC retrofit on 7500 taxis	12.5 million	1.5%	8.4 million
SCR on 26 largest sources	180 million	20%	9 million
TWC retrofit on 1000 LPG buses	2.5 million	0.2%	12.5 million
Moving 20 factories	9.8 million	0.1%	9.8 million

Note: * = lower range.

the given sequence, SO_2 concentrations could be brought down by about 43 per cent, approaching the target but not quite meeting it. The annual costs would be about RMB400 million.

The NO_x action plan

The following control options for NO_x reduction were analysed in a similar fashion as those for SO_2:

- low NO_x burners (LNBs) in large point sources (combined with over-fire air (OFA));
- selective non-catalytic reduction (SNCR) in large point sources;
- selective catalytic reduction (SCR) in large point sources;
- retrofit of three-way catalytic converters (TWC) on taxis; and
- retrofit of TWC on LPG buses.

In addition, several of the options analysed under SO_2 will also reduce NO_x emissions.

Without going into the same details as for the SO_2 analyses, the main results of the development of the NO_x action plan are given in Table 6.7 and Figure 6.5.

The analysis shows that even as implementing the suggested control options will reduce the NO_x concentrations in control Guangzhou substantially, it does not come close to attaining the NO_x concentration target.

It may be noted that the most effective control options are those associated with the large point sources, not those associated with road traffic. It should

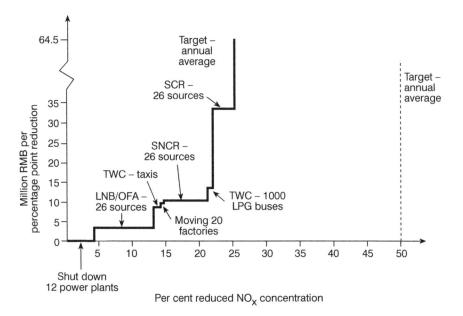

Figure 6.5 *Cost curve, NO$_x$ control options*

then further be noted that as the action plan was developed to look at improving the air quality situation in the short term (by 2001), the more effective long term control options related to road vehicles were not considered. Such options include the introduction of TWCs and improved engine technologies in the entire car fleet, which after a period of some ten years would result in more substantial NO$_x$ reductions.

It should also be noted that the NO$_x$ target concentration, based on the air quality standards of China at the time, was $50\mu g/m^3$ measured as annual average of total NO$_x$. This is a very strict target, much stricter than those used in, for example, the European Union or the US. It is currently being reconsidered.

CONCLUSIONS

Authorities attempting to reduce air pollution are unlikely to choose the most cost-effective measures unless a systematic assessment is undertaken and actions are selected at least partly on this basis. As illustrated in the examples presented in this chapter, it is possible to conduct relatively comprehensive assessments and develop action plans even in cities that do not have all of the data that would be desirable. Moreover, the differences in cost-effectiveness can be very large, even among options that may all seem superficially attractive. For a city that is serious about controlling air pollution, the costs of an assessment are likely to be quickly offset by the savings from choosing the more cost-effective measures.

Not all urban centres can be expected to carry out assessments or develop action plans as detailed in those summarized above. The same logic can usually be applied, however, and the process of carrying out this type of exercise can help to identify the most important information gaps.

NOTES

1   The leading partner institution on the Guangzhou side was the Guangzhou Research Institute for Environmental Protection (GRIEP). The main participants at GRIEP were Wu Zhengqi (Director and Project Coordinator), Fan Changzhong, Luo Jiahai and Gong Hui. On the Norwegian side the project was coordinated by the NILU (Norsk Institut for Luftforskning – Norwegian Institute for Air Research) with Steinar Larssen as project coordinator. Participating Norwegian institutions were the ECON Centre for Economic Analysis, the Centre for International Climate and Environmental Research and the Institute for Energy Technology.
2   Ideally, the concentration reduction potential should be calculated in terms of the total reduction in the exposure of the population (calculated as reduction in concentration x inhabitants affected). Due to time constraints related to the final deadline of the project, this calculation of concentration and exposure reduction potential had to be simplified somewhat.
3   The regional background concentration of the area (non-urban concentration) is naturally included as a part of the urban SO_2 concentration. The regional background is considered to be unaffected by the control options analysed.

REFERENCES

Aarhus, K, Larssen, S, Annan, K, Vennemo, H, Lindhjem, H, Henriksen, J F and Sandvei, K (2000) *Guangzhou Air Quality Action Plan 2001*, NORAD project CHN013, ECON Report 9/2000, Guangzhou Air Quality Management and Planning System, Norsk Institut for Luftforskning, Norway

EU (1998) Common Position (EC) No 57/98, adopted by the Council on 24 September with a view to adoption of Council Directive 98/_/EC relating to limit values for sulphur dioxide, nitrogen dioxide and oxides of nitrogen, particulate matter and lead in ambient air (98/C360/04), *Official Journal of the European Communities*, C360/99

Faiz, A, Weaver, C S and Walsh, MP (1996) *Air Pollution from Motor Vehicles: Standards and Technologies for Controlling Emissions*, World Bank, Washington, DC

Larssen, S (1998) 'Monitoring networks and air quality management systems' in J Fenger et al (eds) *Urban Air Pollution: European Aspects*, Kluwer Academic Publishers, Dordrecht

Larssen, S (ed) (2000) *Guangzhou Air Quality Management and Planning System*, NORAD project CHN013, Norsk Institut for Luftforskning, Norway

Larssen, S and Helmis, C (1998) 'Quality assurance and quality control' in J Fenger et al (eds) *Urban Air Pollution: European Aspects*, Kluwer Academic Publishers, Dordrecht

Mishan, E J (1988) *Cost Benefit Analysis*, Fourth Edition, Unwin Hyman, London

Ostro, B (1992) *Estimating the Health and Economic Effects of Air Pollution in Jakarta: A Preliminary Assessment*, paper presented at the Fourth Annual Meeting of the International Society of Environmental Epidemiology, August, Cuernavaca, Mexico

Ostro, B (1994) *Estimating the Health Effects of Air Pollutants: A Method with an Application to Jakarta*, Policy Research Working Paper 1301, World Bank, Washington, DC

Shah, J J and Nagpal, T (eds) (1997a) *Urban AQMS in Asia, Greater Mumbai Report*, World Bank Technical Paper No 381, World Bank, Washington, DC

Shah, J J and Nagpal, T (eds) (1997b) *Urban AQMS in Asia, Metro Manila Report*, World Bank Technical Paper No 380, World Bank, Washington, DC

Shah, J J and Nagpal, T (eds) (1997c) *Urban AQMS in Asia, Jakarta Report*, World Bank Technical Paper No 379, World Bank, Washington, DC

Shah, J J and Nagpal, T (eds) (1997d) *Urban AQMS in Asia, Kathmandu Valley Report*, World Bank Technical Paper No 378, World Bank, Washington, DC

Shah, J J, Nagpal, T and Brandon, C J (eds) (1997) *Urban AQMS in Asia: Guidebook*, World Bank, Washington, DC

US EPA (1997) *Federal Register*, vol 62, no 138, pp38651–38701

WHO (1992) *Urban Air Pollution in Megacities of the World*, World Health Organization/United Nations Environment Programme/Blackwell Publishers, Cambridge, MA

WHO (1995) *Update and Revision of the Air Quality Guidelines for Europe*, Meeting of the Working Group on Classical Air Pollutants, Bilthoven, The Netherlands, 11–14 October, 1994, WHO Regional Office for Europe (EUR/ICP/EHAZ 94 05/PB01), Copenhagen

7

Indoor Air Pollution

Sumeet Saksena and Kirk R Smith

ABSTRACT

This chapter examines the potential impact of indoor air pollution on health in developing countries, with a particular emphasis on exposure to particulates. It begins by reviewing the evidence on the emissions, concentrations and populations exposed to indoor air pollution from traditional cooking fuels. Given the magnitudes involved, and despite considerable uncertainty, the chapter argues that the scales of exposure and health effects are likely to be large. The chapter presents the emerging scientific evidence that supports the numerous anecdotal accounts relating high biomass smoke levels to important health effects. These are principally acute respiratory infection in children, and chronic obstructive lung disease, adverse pregnancy outcomes and lung cancer in women. The chapter concludes that more research is sorely needed, however, before reliable estimates can be made of the burden of disease associated with indoor air pollution (rough estimates indicate it to be one of the largest single risk factors for mortality – roughly 6 per cent globally) and how much ill-health would be reduced by smoke reduction activities such as the promotion of improved stoves.

INTRODUCTION

Power production, urbanization and rapid industrialization have generally been regarded as the primary causes of deteriorating air quality. Policy-makers and environmental managers tend to ignore the role of small sources of air pollution, particularly when they do not contribute substantially to ambient emissions. Small sources can be very important, however, when they have a high exposure effectiveness, defined as the fraction of the emitted pollution from a source that actually enters people's breathing zones.

The health damage produced by air pollution is dependent on the dose received by the population in question (see Chapter 1). Because dose is difficult to determine for large numbers of people, however, air pollution studies have tended to emphasize exposure, which is usually assumed to be closely proportional to dose. In practice, a surrogate for exposure – ambient concentration – has actually been measured in most instances. This has been done, for example, by placing monitoring instruments on the roofs of public buildings in urban areas. This practice assumes that overall ambient concentration is well characterized by the particular choice of places and times that measurements are made, and that actual human exposures nearby are proportional to the ambient concentration so determined. In fact, a relatively small fraction of time is spent outdoors in developed country cities, where the bulk of air pollution measurement and control efforts have taken place. The air quality in indoor environments where people spend most of their time is influenced by outdoor pollution, but also by indoor sources (Smith, 2002a).

Indoor exposures to air pollution are substantially larger than indicated by outdoor concentrations when there are large indoor sources, such as open fuel or tobacco burning. Globally, the most important indoor sources relate to the use of traditional household solid fuels, biomass and coal. These play a vital role in the developing world where more than 2 billion people rely on them to meet the majority of their energy needs. These fuels are often obtained from the local natural environment on which people also depend for food crops and grazing for their animals. In simple stoves, however, these fuels produce rather large emissions of health-damaging pollutants.

The term 'traditional fuels' refers principally to biomass fuels used mainly for household energy, including wood, charcoal, agricultural residues and animal waste. In some countries, China most prominently, coal also plays an important role. It is estimated that such fuels account for roughly 20–35 per cent of the total energy consumption in developing countries (UNDP, 2000). In India, for example, it is estimated that about 62 per cent of households use firewood and agricultural waste, 15 per cent use animal wastes and 3 per cent use coal or coke (GOI, 1992).

When people are no longer able to rely on an abundance of good quality firewood but cannot afford or do not have access to fossil fuels, they are gradually forced to exercise care and frugality in the use of a variety of lower quality fuels – to move down what is called the 'household energy ladder'. As a result, a new equilibrium in fuel use is eventually reached. Even if people are still able to meet their household energy needs, there is no question that for many it represents a lowering in the quality of their daily lives.

Figure 7.1 illustrates the evolutionary path for cooking fuels and stoves in most developing countries. In some cases, changes in income or the availability of other resources may force some groups back down this path but, in general, people prefer, if possible, to move upwards. Although it is useful for describing large scale historical movements in fuel use, individual households often straddle two or more steps on the ladder (rely on two or more types of fuel) and may shift fuel use up or down according to the time of year, the cost of fuel and other parameters.

In summary, biofuels are among the most important fuels globally in terms of the number of people affected. In energy content, they are the most

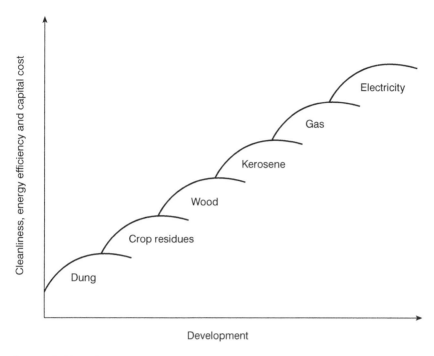

Source: Smith et al, 1994

Figure 7.1 *The generic household energy ladder*

important fuels in many poor countries, although second to fossil fuels on a global basis. They are used principally by households for cooking and space heating. Furthermore, they are likely to remain important in many developing countries for many decades to come.

CONCENTRATIONS AND EXPOSURES

Although there are many hundreds of separate chemical agents that have been identified in biofuel smoke, the four most emphasized pollutants are particulates, carbon monoxide, polycyclic organic matter and formaldehyde. Unfortunately, relatively little monitoring has been done in rural and poor urban indoor environments in a manner that is statistically rigorous. The results nevertheless are striking (Table 7.1). The concentrations found are 10–100 times higher than typical health-related standards/guidelines. The rest of the discussion will be restricted to particulate matter (PM) because of data gaps regarding other pollutants, and because PM is probably the best single indicator of potential harm.

There are few micro-levels studies that have attempted to measure total exposure levels in communities using biofuels. The first study that measured levels of pollutants in various micro-environments (cooking and non-cooking, indoor and outdoor) and the time spent in each of these by different population

Table 7.1 *Typical concentration levels of TSP matter indoors from biofuel combustion measured through area and personal sampling*

Country	Year	Sample size	Conditions	Concentration ($\mu g/m^3$)
I Area concentrations				
Papua New Guinea	1968	9	overnight, floor level	5200
	1974	6	overnight, sitting level	1300
Kenya	1971–72	8	overnight, highlands/ lowlands	4000/800
	1988	64	24-hour, thatched/ iron roof	1300/1500 (R)
India	1982	64	30-minute wood/ dung/charcoal	15,800/18,300/ 5500
	1988	390	cooking, 0.7 metre ceiling	4000/21,000
	1992	145	cooking/non-cooking/ living	5600/820/630
	1994	61	24-hour, agricultural residue/wood	2800/2000 (I)
	1995	50	Breakfast/lunch/dinner	850/1250/1460 (I)
	1996	136	Urban, cooking/ sleeping	2860/880 (I)
Nepal	1986	17	2 hours	4400 (I)
China	1986	64		2570
	1987	4	8 hours	10,900 (I)
	1988	9	2 houses, 12 hours	2900
	1988	12	4 houses, dung	3000 (I)
	1990	15	Dung, winter/summer	1670/830 (I)
	1991		Straw, average summer/winter, kitchen/living	1650/610/1570(I)
	1991		Single storey/double storey hourouses	80/170
	1993	4		1060 (I)
Gambia	1988	36	24-hour, dry/wet season	2000/2100 (I)
Zimbabwe	1990	40	2 hours	1300 (I)
Brazil	1992	11	2–3 hours, traditional/ improved stove	1100/90 (I)
Guatemala	1993	44	24-hour, traditional/ improved stove	1200/530 (I)
	1996	18	24-hour, traditional/ improved stove	720/190 (I), 520/90 (I)
	1996	43	24-hour, traditional/ improved stove	870/150 (R)
South Africa	1993	20	12-hour, kitchen/ bedroom	1720/1020
Mexico	1995	31	9 hours	335/439 (R)/(I)

II Personal monitoring

India	1983	65	4 villages	6800
	1987	165	8 villages	3700
	1987	44	2 villages	3600
	1988	129	5 villages	4700
	1991	95	winter/summer/ monsoon	6800/5400/4800
	1996	40	two urban slums, infants, 24-hour	400/520 (I)
Nepal	1986	49	2 villages	2000
	1990	40	Traditional/improved stove	8200/3000
Zambia	1992	184	4-hour, urban, wood/charcoal	470/210 (R)
Ghana	1993	43	3-hour, urban, wood/charcoal	590/340 (R)
South Africa	1993	15	12-hour, children, winter/summer	2370/290

Notes: Unless noted otherwise, figures refer to total suspended particulates (TSP, also sometimes referred to as suspended particulate matter or SPM).
I = inhalable particulate matter (less than 10–15 microns).
R = respirable particulate matter (less than 2.5–5 microns).
Source: Smith, 1996

groups was conducted in a rural hilly area of India. The study concluded (see Table 7.2) that the daily exposure levels of women and children far exceed comparable Indian or international standards and those of young people and men (Saksena et al, 1992), and that cooking was the major contributor to daily exposure for women and children.

A recent study in Kenya confirmed that adult women (age 16–50) experience extremely high daily exposures to PM less than 10 micrometres in aerodynamic diameter (PM_{10}). Mean levels as high as 4.9mg/m^3 were observed as compared to 1mg/m^3 for males of the same age group (Ezzati et al, 2000). In Bolivia, a study by Albalak et al (1999) indicated that daily exposures of women to PM_{10} were 0.47–0.63mg/m^3, depending on whether food was cooked inside or outside. In Guatemala, measurements of $PM_{2.5}$ during cooking sessions indicated average levels of 5.3 and 1.9mg/m^3 for open fires and improved stoves respectively (Naeher et al, 2000).

The few studies that enable a comparison of daily levels across various fuel groups confirm the concept of the energy ladder (as one moves up the ladder, the cleanliness, efficiency and convenience of the fuels tend to increase, along with their costs), as indicated in Table 7.3.

An estimate of exposure on a global level has ascribed approximately 77 per cent of the global exposure to particulates to indoor environments in the developing world (WHO, 1997). Such estimates are based on the pollutant levels (concentrations) considered typical in different micro-environments, estimates of the time spent by various population groups in these micro-environments, and the size of these groups. Reliable estimates would require a good database

Table 7.2 *Mean daily integrated exposure to TSP (mg/m³) in a rural hilly area of India*

Season	Women	Children	Young people	Men
Winter	1.96	1.04	0.79	0.71
Summer	1.13	0.54	0.33	0.25

Note: Daily Indian ambient standard for residential areas is 0.1mg/m³; the WHO guideline was 0.10–0.15mg/m³.
Source: Saksena et al, 1992

of time-activity patterns linked to location-specific exposure estimates. This does not exist at the present time. Indoor exposure estimates depend heavily on the relatively few surveys that have been conducted in rural areas. However, if these results are representative, the overall health burden is likely to be extremely high.

HEALTH EFFECTS

The total human exposure to many important pollutants is much more substantial in the homes of the poor in developing countries than in the outdoor air of cities in the developed world because of the high concentrations and the large populations involved. It is, however, the outdoor problem that has received the vast majority of attention in the form of air pollution research and control efforts (Smith, 1993). As a result, it has been necessary to extrapolate from urban studies to estimate what the health effects might be in biomass-using households. In recent years, however, there have been a number of studies that directly focus on these households and which generally confirm what has been extrapolated (Bruce et al, 2000; Smith et al, 2000; Smith, 2000). There follows some brief summaries of the major health effects. It must be remembered that the quality of these studies is not as high as desirable, mainly because of inappropriate choices of exposure and health outcome indicators, poor study design, weak statistical foundations and a failure to consider certain confounding factors.

Acute respiratory infection in children (ARI)

ARI, particularly as an acute lower respiratory infection (ALRI) such as pneumonia, is one of the chief killers of children in developing countries. At about 4 million deaths per year, it now exceeds deaths from diarrhoea (Murray and Lopez, 1996). ARI is known to be enhanced by exposures to urban air pollutants and indoor environmental tobacco smoke at levels of pollution some 10–30 times less than typically found in village homes.

Some of the most suggestive studies available were undertaken in Nepal, Zimbabwe and Gambia. A Nepal study examined approximately 240 rural children under two years of age each week for six months for incidence of moderate and severe ARI (Pandey et al, 1989). They found a strong relationship

Table 7.3 *Estimated daily exposures to PM$_{10}$ (mg/m^3) from cooking fuel along energy ladder in two Asian cities*

Fuel	Pune, India	Beijing, China
Biomass	0.71–1.08	
Coal (vented)		0.10–0.15
Kerosene	0.1–0.15	
Liquefied petroleum gas	0.02	0.06
National ambient standard (for residential areas)	0.10	0.15

Source: Adapted from Smith et al, 1994

between the maternally reported number of hours per day the children stayed by the fire and the incidence of moderate and severe cases. In Zimbabwe, 244 children under three reporting at hospitals with ARI were compared with 500 similar children reporting at clinics (Collings et al, 1990). The presence of an open wood fire was found to be a significant ARI risk factor. In a study of 500 children in Gambia, girls under five carried on their mothers' backs during cooking (in smoky cooking huts) were found to have a six times greater risk of ARI, a substantially higher risk factor than parental smoking. There was no significant risk, however, in young boys (probably because they are kept for shorter periods near the fire) (Armstrong and Campbell, 1991).

A study in Buenos Aires (Cerqueiro et al, 1990) used a matched case-control method to identify risk factors for ALRI in 670 children. The results of the study indicated a high risk from indoor contaminants.

Four hundred children under five years of age in South Kerala, India were studied to identify risk factors for severe pneumonia. The cases were in-patients with severe pneumonia as ascertained by WHO criteria, while controls were out-patients with non-severe ARI. There was no association with the presence of an improved 'smokeless' cook-stove in the children's homes (Shah et al, 1994). This is consistent with other studies in India that often show no significant difference in indoor pollution in households with and without improved stoves (Ramakrishna et al, 1989). O'Dempsey et al (1996) investigated possible risk factors for pneumococcal disease among children living in a rural area of the Gambia. A prospective case-control study was conducted. The study indicated that there is an increased risk of pneumococcal diseases associated with children being carried on their mothers' backs during cooking.

Overall, the studies conducted to date are extremely suggestive and, with a few exceptions, reasonably consistent. Being quantitative, they can be used to calculate health effects (see below). They do not fulfil all the strict scientific requirements for demonstrating causality because ARI has so many other risk factors for which it is difficult to account in studies that observe pre-existing differences in exposure conditions. In particular, if biomass fuel use is associated with poverty, which is itself associated with other risk factors, then assigning risk to pollution from biomass fires can be problematic. Randomized trials are needed in which exposure-reduction technologies, for example, improved fuels or stoves, are applied to half the households in a population, which are then followed to see if ARI rates diverge. In this way one can be fairly certain that other ARI risk factors, for example socio-economic or nutritional, do not vary between groups using different types of fuels or stoves. Until such studies are conducted it is necessary to relay the results of less rigorously designed studies.

Chronic obstructive pulmonary disease and cor pulmonale

Chronic obstructive pulmonary disease (COPD), for which tobacco smoking is the major risk factor remaining in the developed countries, is known to be an outcome of excessive air pollution exposure. It is difficult to study because the exposures that cause the illness may occur many years before the symptoms are seen. Nevertheless, studies in Nepal (Pandey, 1984) and India (Malik, 1985; Behera and Jindal, 1991) led the investigators to conclude that non-smoking women who have cooked on biomass stoves for many years exhibit a higher prevalence of this condition than might be expected for similar women who have had less use of biomass stoves. In rural Nepal, nearly 15 per cent of non-smoking women (20 years and older) had chronic bronchitis, a high rate for non-smokers.

Cor pulmonale (heart disease secondary to chronic lung disease) has been found to be prevalent and to develop earlier than average in non-smoking women who cook with biomass in India (Padmavati and Arora, 1976) and Nepal (Pandey et al, 1988).

A population-based cross-sectional survey was conducted to determine the prevalence of chronic bronchitis and associated risk factors in an urban area of Southern Brazil, where 1053 subjects aged 40 years and over were interviewed. High levels of indoor air pollution were found to be associated with an increased (nearly doubled) prevalence of the disease (Menezes et al, 1994).

Cancer

There are many chemicals in biomass smoke that are known to cause cancer (Cooper, 1980). In the 1970s, based on a small study in Kenya, it was thought that naso-pharyngeal cancer might be associated with biomass smoke (Clifford, 1972) but more recent studies in Malaysia (Armstrong et al, 1978) and Hong Kong (Yu et al, 1985) have failed to confirm this. Based on risk extrapolations from animal studies, lung cancer, which might be expected to be common in biomass-using areas, is relatively rare (Koo et al, 1983). Indeed, some of the lowest lung cancer rates in the world are found in rural non-smoking women in developing countries. This is something of an anomaly, and can only be partly explained by poor health records. A recent study in Japan (Sobue et al, 1990), on the other hand, found that women cooking with straw or woodfuel when they were 30 years old have an 80 per cent increased chance of having lung cancer in later life (cancer, as in the case of chronic lung disease, takes many years after exposure to develop).

Compared to biomass, there are many studies of the air pollution levels and health impacts of cooking with coal on open stoves, almost all undertaken and published in China where coal use for cooking is common (Hong, 1991). A range of effects is found, including quite strong associations with lung cancer (Smith and Liu, 1994). Even in China, however, biomass use is much more prevalent, and yet has not received adequate scientific and policy attention.

Tuberculosis

One of the most disturbing implications of recent research is that wood smoke might be associated with tuberculosis (TB). A large scale survey (89,000 households) in India found that women over 20 years old in households using biofuels were nearly three times more likely to report having TB than those in households using cleaner fuels, even after accounting for a range of socio-economic factors (Mishra et al, 1999a). A study with clinically confirmed TB in Lucknow, India found a similar risk, but was not able to correct for socio-economic factors (Gupta et al, 1997).

Adverse pregnancy outcomes

Low birthweight, a chronic problem in developing countries, is associated with a number of health problems in early infancy as well as other negative outcomes such as neonatal death. Several risk factors are associated with low birthweight, most notably poor nutrition. Since active smoking by the mother during pregnancy is a known risk factor and exposure to smoke is suspected, there is also reason to suspect biomass smoke as it contains many of the same pollutants. Carbon monoxide, which studies in Guatemala (Dary et al, 1981) and India (Behera et al, 1988) found in substantial amounts in the blood of women cooking with biomass, is an air pollutant of particular concern. Another study in India found that pregnant women cooking over open biomass stoves had an almost 50 per cent bigger chance of stillbirth (Mavalankar, 1991).

Blindness

A case-control study in India found an excess cataract risk of about 80 per cent among people using biofuels (Mohan et al, 1989). Cataracts are the main cause of blindness in India and are known to be caused by wood smoke in laboratory animals. The same large family survey mentioned above found a somewhat lower rate (77 per cent) for partial blindness in adults living in Indian households with clean fuels, and a significant difference for total blindness in women (Mishra et al, 1999b).

HEALTH IMPACTS

Based on extrapolations of health effects in developed countries, WHO has estimated that 2.7–3 million premature deaths (5–6 per cent of annual global deaths) occur due to outdoor and indoor air pollution (WHO, 1997). A recent evaluation of the national burden of disease in India from indoor air pollution relied only on studies done in biomass-using households (many of them are discussed above) instead of trying to extrapolate from developed-country urban settings that have been the basis of most air pollution health effects studies (Smith, 1998). Using national census data on the distribution of biomass use, the study estimated that some 400,000–600,000 premature deaths per year among Indian women and children under five can be attributed to indoor air pollution. (Data were too poor to estimate the lower risks experienced by men and older children.) Extrapolating the Indian estimates to the entire South Asia region would indicate some 500,000–700,000 premature deaths each year from indoor air pollution among women and young children alone. Extrapolation worldwide might indicate a total of 1.2–1.6 million, with a large number in sub-Saharan Africa.

Although based on the best available evidence, it is emphasized that such estimates must be considered preliminary. Too little effort has gone into conducting either the health effects or exposure assessment studies in biomass-using populations. Nevertheless, it seems clear that the potential magnitude is substantial.[1]

Knowledge Gaps and Necessary Research

A high research priority is to conduct epidemiological studies to identify the relationships between ARI, indoor air quality (biomass smoke, tobacco smoke), nutritional status, other infections, family/household composition, variables, and so on (Smith, 2002b).

Possible research strategies for epidemiological studies have been identified and these include the following:

- Case-control studies to establish relationships and identify dose–response and dose–effect relationships; some studies have been done but more are needed.
- Studies of 'natural experiments' in which incidence rates of episodes might be examined longitudinally in relation to such changes as introducing stoves with chimneys in dwellings previously lacking chimneys.
- Randomized intervention studies in which health status is assessed with and without interventions such as improved stoves.

Intervention studies are suitable only for health effects that occur relatively quickly after exposure. The highest priority for intervention studies would thus seem to be:

- ARI in young children; and
- adverse pregnancy outcomes for women exposed during pregnancy.

Since the association of COPD and biomass smoke is fairly well established and lung cancer is not a major problem among non-smoking women in most developing countries, the highest priority for case-control studies would seem to be:

- TB in adult women; and
- heart disease in adult women.

TB is of special interest because it is increasing in South Asia due to the growing HIV epidemic. Heart disease, which is one of the chief outcomes of urban air pollution studies in developed countries, has apparently never been studied in biomass-using households.

All such studies, of course, should meet accepted scientific standards for quality control and ethical conduct. In order to maximize scarce resources, research should be linked where possible to existing research projects that have already gathered some of the crucial information on ARI or other outcomes in the target groups (examples include vitamin A deficiency and family planning projects).

Work is needed to improve the quality of existing data and to facilitate the collection of new data. The most accurate available indicator of indoor air pollution is personal and area monitoring for respirable suspended particulates (RSP). Further work is required, however, to improve the capacity to simply and quickly assess exposure to indoor air pollution. It is difficult to assess exposure in children aged from two to five years with existing methods; time-weighted area monitoring might be the best choice.

INTERVENTIONS

This is a two-fold challenge facing most developing societies attempting to sustainably manage the biomass energy transition. First, there is a need to find sustainable means to harvest biofuels for the needs of that majority of humanity now relying upon them. Second, there is a need to develop high grade biomass fuels (liquid and gaseous) that can meet development requirements, and to improve the efficiency, controllability and cleanliness of end-use devices.

Fuels

In the past, rural development was typically accompanied by a transition from traditional biofuels to fossil fuels, particularly kerosene, diesel oil and LPG (liquefied petroleum gas). In recent years, however, it has often been concluded that the cost and insecurity of petroleum supplies will delay or deny this transition in many of the now-developing countries. Given that the international price of petroleum is lower than it has been for many decades, however, it is no longer clear that this conclusion is valid. Furthermore, reserving sufficient clean-burning gaseous and liquid fuels for household applications where pollution has such important health implications would seem an appropriate policy objective.

Although substantial, the cost of importing sufficient clean fossil fuels for South Asian households would not necessarily be prohibitive (Parikh et al, 1999). For example, it has been estimated that the petroleum demand for powering the South Asian light vehicle (mainly car) fleet will grow at an average annual rate of 7.6 per cent until 2020 (WEC, 1998). If the annual growth rate were lowered slightly to 6 per cent, by 2020 the difference in vehicle fuel use would amount to some 40 million litres a day of kerosene equivalent. This quantity could supply most of the region's current biomass-using households and entail no more oil imports than are now being planned for vehicles. Recognizing that directing this fuel solely to households is no easy task, it is nevertheless clear that the issue is to a great degree one of social priorities.

In the short term, however, it appears that the economic and logistical barriers to meeting rural energy needs solely by fossil fuels will be unsurmountable. This implies that biofuels will have a continuing role for many decades and must be taken seriously by policy-makers if the behaviour of the entire national energy system is to be understood and manipulated. If biofuels are to provide the type of energy services previously accomplished by the petroleum fuels, there must be substantial changes in the form and use of these fuels. So dramatic are these changes that it is appropriate to call them part of the post-biofuel transition or, more accurately, the post-traditional biofuel transition. This transition is occurring at every stage of the biofuel cycle, from harvesting through conversion to end use (Smith, 1986).

At the production stage, a change is occurring from unplanned and unscientific practices of gathering biofuel to sustainable harvesting. At the conversion stage, a number of processes are becoming available to upgrade the relatively low grade natural solid biofuels into high grade solid, liquid and gaseous fuels that can fuel a wide range of tasks beyond the basic necessities of cooking and space heating that biofuel now caters for. More importantly, equipment is now being developed to accomplish these conversions at the village and household scales. Examples are biogas and producer gas devices, alcohol fermentation and charcoal manufacture. Some of these conversion processes have the additional advantage that they remove the most polluting step out of the household to a village or otherwise more centralized location. This can greatly reduce individual exposures even if total emissions are not reduced.

With a view to reducing the pressure on forests and other biomass resources, countries such as India and Pakistan are trying to promote coal as a cooking fuel. Such a move has its merits and demerits. Many studies in China and South Africa have indicated that household coal use leads to significant health hazards. China has the highest lung cancer rate for non-smoking women who use coal. Emissions from coal contain the very same pollutants as biomass emissions; in addition, they contain toxic substances such as sulphur, arsenic and fluorine (Parikh et al, 1999).

Stoves

In the short and medium term, improving the use of biofuels seems to be the only feasible option for many households. Until recently, most stove research and implementation programmes considered fuel savings to be the primary goal. The relationships between the various parameters that govern stove performance are complex and surprisingly ill understood. Nevertheless, it seems likely that research can lead to the development of cooking systems that are so efficient that overall exposure can be reduced while ensuring an optimal thermal performance and social acceptability.

Large scale acceptance of improved stoves would require a concerted effort on the part of local organizations as well as governments to mass produce them in an appropriate manner and overcome the social resistance to change. Many of the most important barriers to new stove introductions are not technical but relate to social and marketing questions (Smith, 1987). Currently, nearly all the improved stove designs in South Asia are aimed either at increasing fuel efficiency or at removing smoke from the house via a chimney or flue. Some try to accomplish both goals. Few, however, attempt to modify the combustion conditions in such a way that both efficiency and low emissions are achieved (see Chapter 1). From a health perspective, providing a flue to take the smoke from the room is often sufficient. In urban areas, however, such measures are likely to have less of an impact on exposure, and achieving low emissions is more important.

Unfortunately, experience with the Indian large scale improved stove programme indicates that locally made stoves have quite short lifetimes in households, perhaps less than one year on average (Kishore and Ramana, 2002). Preliminary cost–benefit analysis in India, on the other hand, indicates that it is difficult to justify many improved stoves on health grounds unless lifetimes exceed ten years (Smith, 1998). Such lifetimes seem likely only with stoves manufactured with durable materials. One approach is to manufacture the crucial combustion chamber components using high quality materials under good quality control, ship them to the households and have the householders construct the outer, less critical, parts of the stoves using local materials. This is the approach taken by the highly successful Chinese improved stove programme, which has introduced more than 150 million improved stoves since 1980 (Smith et al, 1993).

Housing improvements

In addition to changing the fuel or the stove, another option for reducing air pollutant levels is to improve the ventilation where the fuel is being used. The easiest solution in principle would be to move the cooking activity outdoors and for the stove to be located downwind from the cook or other persons nearby.

If biofuels are to be in use in rural areas for many years, then consideration should be given to changing the designs for new rural housing units to improve ventilation in the kitchen area. Although it may seem obvious that such ventilation ought to be included in new designs, there are many instances where it is not. Some designs promoted by the rural housing extension programmes of some of the major Asian countries, for example, do not explicitly include such features (Smith, 1987).

Improved awareness

Although scientific and medical experts seem to realize that indoor air pollution is potentially a significant problem, the people who are really affected by it – the poor women of developing countries – do not seem to be aware at all of the hazards they and their children face. Two surveys – one in Jakarta, Indonesia and another in Accra, Ghana – highlighted the fact that such households rank indoor air pollution as one of the lowest priority problems in comparison to other problems such as water, waste and pests (Surjadi et al, 1994; Benneh et al, 1993). Even their willingness to pay for improvements in indoor air quality was found to be low. This was found to be true across all income groups.

In South Asia there is perhaps a slightly higher awareness of the potential risks. A household survey conducted in North and South India indicated that only 17–24 per cent of the people think that indoor air pollution is not a problem (Ramakrishna, 1988). Between 35–52 per cent of the households responded that they had not taken any ameliorative measures. Although people are obviously aware of the relative smokiness of various fuels, they did not appear to make conscious efforts to procure and use less smoky fuels. In fact, many people actually see benefits in the smoke, such as repelling mosquitoes and preserving the roof. Clearly, there is a need for better education, awareness and risk communication programmes.

CONCLUSIONS

Given the enormous emissions, concentrations and populations involved in the use of traditional cooking fuels, the scale of exposures and health effects is likely to be large. There is growing scientific evidence to support the numerous anecdotal accounts that relate high biomass smoke levels to important health effects. These are, principally, ARI in children, COPD, adverse pregnancy outcomes and lung cancer in women. Of late, there are indications that tuberculosis, asthma and blindness may be associated with indoor air pollution. More research is sorely needed, however, before reliable estimates can be made about how much of the global burden of disease can be attributed to indoor air pollution (rough estimates indicate it to be one of the largest single risk factors for mortality, at approximately 6 per cent) and how much ill-health would be reduced by smoke-reduction activities such as the promotion of improved stoves.

The key areas for intervention are developing high grade biomass fuels, improving stove designs and dissemination approaches, improving housing and improving awareness and education.

NOTE

1   The WHO organized a large scale comparative risk assessment of about 30 major risk factors worldwide, and these were published in *The World Health Report 2002*. Separate estimates of the health effects of indoor and outdoor air pollution were made as part of this assessment (WHO, 2002).

REFERENCES

Albalak, R, Keeler, G J, Frisancho, A R and Haber, M (1999) 'Assessment of PM[10] concentrations from domestic biomass fuel combustion in two rural Bolivian highland villages'in *Environmental Science and Technology*, vol 33, no 15, pp2505–2509

Armstrong, R W et al (1978) 'Self-specific environments associated with nasopharyngeal carcinoma in Selangor, Malaysia' in *Social Science and Medicine*, vol 12, no 3D–4D, pp149–156

Armstrong, J R M and Campbell, H (1991) 'Indoor air pollution exposure and lower respiratory infection in young Gambian children' in *International Journal of Epidemiology*, vol 20, no 2, pp424–428

Behera, D, Dash, S and Malik, S K (1988) 'Blood carboxyhaemoglobin levels following acute exposure to smoke of biomass fuel' in *Indian Journal of Medical Research*, vol 88, pp522–524

Behera, D and Jindal, S K (1991) 'Respiratory symptoms in Indian women using domestic cooking fuels' in *Chest,* vol 100, no 2, pp385–388

Benneh, G, Songsore, J, Nabila, J S, Amuzu, A T, Tutu, K A, Yangyuoru, Y and McGranahan, G (1993) *Environmental Problems and the Urban Household in the Greater Accra Metropolitan Area (GAMA), Ghana*, Stockholm Environment Institute, Stockholm

Bruce, N, Perez-Padilla, R and Albalak, R (2000) 'Indoor air pollution in developing countries: a major environmental and public health challenge' in *Bulletin of the World Health Organization*, vol 78, no 9, pp1078–1092

Cerqueiro, M C, Murtagh, P, Halac, A, Avila, M and Weissenbacher, M (1990) 'Epidemiologic risk factors for children with acute lower respiratory tract infection in Buenos Aires, Argentina: a matched case-control study' in *Reviews of Infectious Diseases*, vol 12, no 8, ppS1021–S1028

Clifford, P (1972) 'Carcinogens in the nose and throat: nasopharyngeal carcinoma in Kenya' in *Proceedings of the Royal Society of Medicine*, vol 65, no 8, pp682–686

Collings, D A, Sithole, S D and Martin, K S (1990) 'Indoor woodsmoke pollution causing lower respiratory disease in children' in *Tropical Doctor*, vol 20, no 4, pp151–155

Cooper, J A (1980) 'Environmental impact of residential wood combustion emission and its implications' in *Journal of Air Pollution Control Association*, vol 30, pp855–861

Dary, O, Pineda, O and Belizan, J M (1981) 'Carbon monoxide contamination in dwellings in poor rural areas of Guatemala' in *Bulletin of Environmental Contamination and Toxicology*, vol 26, no 1, pp24–30

Ezzati, M, Saleh, H and Kammen, D M (2000) 'The contributions of emissions and spatial microenvironments to exposure to indoor air pollution from biomass combustion in Kenya' in *Environmental Health Perspectives*, vol 108, no 9, pp833–839

GOI (1992) *Housing and Amenities*, Occasional Paper No 5, Census of India, 1991, Government of India, New Delhi

Gupta, B N, Mathur, N, Mahendra, P N et al (1997) 'A study of household environmental risk factors pertaining to respiratory diseases' in *Energy Environment Monitor,* vol 13, no 2, pp61–68

Hong, C J (1991) *Health Aspects of Domestic Use of Biomass and Coal in China*, WHO/PEP 92.3B, World Health Organization, Geneva

Kishore, V V N and Ramana, P V (2002) 'Improved cookstoves in rural India: how improved?' in *Energy,*vol 27, no 1, pp47–63

Koo, L C, Lee, N and Ho, J H (1983) 'Do cooking fuels pose a risk for lung cancer? A case-control study of women in Hong Kong' in *Ecology and Diseases*, vol 2, no 4, pp255–265

Malik, S K (1985) 'Exposure to domestic cooking fuels and chronic bronchitis' in *Indian Journal of Chest Diseases and Allied Sciences*, vol 27, no 3, pp171–174

Mavalankar, D V (1991) 'Levels and risk factors for perinatal mortality in Ahmedabad, India' in *Bulletin of the World Health Organization*, vol 69, no 4, pp435–442

Menezes, A M, Victora, C G and Rigatto, M (1994) 'Prevalence and risk factors for chronic bronchitis in Pelotas, RS, Brazil: a population-based study' in *Thorax*, vol 49, no 12, pp1217–1221

Mishra, V, Retherford, R D and Smith, K R (1999a) 'Biomass cooking fuels and prevalence of tuberculosis in India' in *International Journal of Infectious Diseases*, vol 3, no 3, pp119–129

Mishra, V, Retherford, R D and Smith, K R (1999b) 'Biomass cooking fuels and prevalence of blindness in India' in *Journal of Environmental Medicine*, vol 1, no 4, pp189–199

Mohan, M, Sperduto, R D, Angra, S K et al (1989) 'India–US case-control study of age-related cataracts' in *Archives of Ophthalmology*, vol 197, pp670–676

Murray, C J L and Lopez, A D (1996) *The Global Burden of Disease*, Harvard University Press, Cambridge, MA

Naeher, L P, Smith, K R, Leaderer, B P, Mage, D and Grajeda, R (2000) 'Indoor and outdoor PM[2.5] and CO in high- and low-density Guatemalan villages' in *Journal of Exposure Analysis and Environmental Epidemiology*, vol 10, pp544–551

O'Dempsey, T J, McArdle, T F, Morris, J, Lloyd-Evans, N, Baldeh, I, Laurence, B E, Seeka, O and Greenwood, B M (1996) 'A study of risk factors for pneumococcal disease among children in a rural area of West Africa' in *International Journal of Epidemiology*, vol 25, no 4, pp885–893

Padmavati, S and Arora, S S (1976) 'Sex differences in chronic cor pulmonale in Delhi' in *British Journal of Diseases of the Chest*, vol 70, no 4, pp251–259

Pandey, M R (1984) 'Domestic smoke pollution and chronic bronchitis in a rural community of the hill region of Nepal' in *Thorax*, vol 39, no 5, pp337–339

Pandey, M R (1988) *Chronic Bronchitis and Cor Pulmonale in Nepal*, Mrigendra Medical Trust, Kathmandu

Pandey, M R, Neupane, R P, Gautam, A and Shrestha, I B (1989) 'Domestic smoke pollution and acute respiratory infections in a rural community of the hill region of Nepal' in *Environment International*, vol 15, pp337–340

Parikh, J, Smith, K R and Laxmi, V (1999) 'Indoor air pollution: a reflection on gender bias' in *Economic and Political Weekly*, February, pp539–544

Ramakrishna, J (1988) *Patterns of Domestic Air Pollution in Rural India*, PhD thesis, University of Hawaii, Honolulu

Ramakrishna, J, Durgaprasad, M B and Smith, K R (1989) 'Cooking in India: the impact of improved stoves on indoor air quality' in *Environment International*, vol 15, no 1–6, pp341–352Saksena, S, Prasad, R, Pal, R C and Joshi, V (1992) 'Patterns of daily exposure to TSP and CO in the Garhwal Himalaya' in *Atmospheric Environment*, vol 26A, no 11, pp2125–2134

Shah, N, Ramankutty, V, Premila, P G and Sathy, N (1994) 'Risk factors for severe pneumonia in children in south Kerala: a hospital-based case-control study' in *Journal of Tropical Pediatrics*, vol 40, no 4, pp201–206

Smith, K R (1986) 'The biofuel transition' in *Pacific and Asian Journal of Energy*, vol 1, no 1, pp17–32

Smith, K R (1987) *Biofuels, Air Pollution and Health: A Global Review*, Plenum Press, New York and London

Smith, K R (1993) 'Fuel combustion, air pollution exposure, and health: the situation in developing countries' in *Annual Review of Energy and Environment*, vol 18, pp529–566

Smith, K R (1996) 'Indoor air pollution in developing countries: growing evidence of its role in the global disease burden' in *Proceedings of Indoor Air '96: The 7th International Conference on Indoor Air Quality and Climate*, Institute of Public Health, Tokyo, vol 3, pp33–34

Smith, K R (1998) *Indoor Air Pollution in India: National Health Impacts and the Cost-effectiveness of Intervention*, Indira Gandhi Institute for Development Research, Mumbai

Smith, K R (2000) 'National burden of disease in India from indoor air pollution' in *Proceedings of the National Academy of Sciences*, vol 97, no 24, pp13286–13293

Smith, K R (2002a) 'Place makes the poison' in *Journal of Exposure Analysis and Environmental Epidemiology,* vol 12, no 3, pp167–171

Smith, K R (2002b) 'Indoor air pollution in developing countries: recommendations for research' in *Indoor Air*, vol 12, no 3, pp198–207

Smith, K R et al (1993) '100 million improved stoves in China: how was it done?' in *World Development*, vol 21, no 6, pp941–961

Smith, K R, Apte, M G, Ma, Y Q, Wongsekiarttirat, W and Kulkarni, A (1994) 'Air pollution and the energy ladder in Asian cities' in *Energy*, vol 19, no 5, pp587–600

Smith, K R and Liu, Y (1994) 'Indoor air pollution in developing countries' in J Samet (ed) *The Epidemiology of Lung Cancer*, Marcell Dekker, New York

Smith, K R, Samet, J M, Romieu, I and Bruce, N (2000) 'Indoor air pollution in developing countries and acute lower respiratory infections in children' in *Thorax*, vol 55, no 6, pp518–532

Sobue, T (1990) 'Association of indoor air pollution and lifestyle with lung cancer in Osaka, Japan' in *International Journal of Epidemiology*, vol 19 (Supplement 1), pps62–s66

Surjadi, C, Padhmasutra, L and Wahyuningsih, D et al (1994) *Household Environmental Problems in Jakarta*, Stockholm Environment Institute, Stockholm

UNDP (2000) World Energy Assessment: Energy and the Challenge of Sustainability, *United Nations Development Programme, New York*

WEC (1998) *Global Transport and Energy Development: Scope for Change*, World Energy Council, London

WHO (1997) *Health and Environment in Sustainable Development: Five Years after the Earth Summit,* World Health Organization, Geneva

WHO (2002) *The World Health Report 2002*, World Health Organization, Geneva

Yu, M C et al (1985) 'Epidemiology of nasopharyngeal carcinoma in Malaysia and Hong Kong' in *National Cancer Institute Monograph*, vol 69, pp203–207

8

Vehicle Emissions and Health in Developing Countries

Michael P Walsh

ABSTRACT

Increasing prosperity and population growth in many developing countries are resulting in accelerated growth in vehicle populations and vehicle miles travelled. While most developing countries currently have very few motorized vehicles per capita compared with the Organisation for Economic Co-operation and Development countries, the vehicle population is growing very rapidly. In South and South-East Asia the popularity of motorcycles and scooters (which have highly polluting two-stroke engines) and other characteristics of the vehicle fleet, such as vehicle age and maintenance, fuel type etc, lead to substantially more emissions per kilometre driven than in the developed countries. As most of the current vehicle population is concentrated in the major cities, these cities usually have poor air quality. This can cause serious health problems, especially with the very old, the very young and those with pre-existing respiratory diseases.

Motor vehicles emit large quantities of carbon monoxide, hydrocarbons, nitrogen oxides and toxic substances including fine particles and lead. Each of these, along with secondary by-products such as ozone, can cause adverse effects on health and the environment. However, significant improvements in air quality are being achieved in some developing countries. Taiwan has implemented a motorcycle control programme expected to eliminate new two-stroke motorcycles by about 2003, and to encourage users to convert to electric motorcycles. Singapore has developed one of the pre-eminent land transport planning programmes in the world serving as a model to its neighbours. Sao Paulo, Brazil is also moving forward with tight vehicle standards.

Many developing countries have made or will soon make progress to reduce vehicle emissions as a major source of air pollution in cities. For example, Thailand banned all sales of leaded gasoline in 1996 and China and India followed in 2000. All new cars sold in Brazil, Hong Kong, Singapore, Taiwan, Thailand and South Korea have been required to be equipped with catalytic converters for several years and China, India and the Philippines recently followed suit.

Table 8.1 *The global population in 1950, 1998 and projected population in 2050, in millions*

	1950	1998	2050
World	2,521	5,901	8,909
More developed regions	813	1,182	1,155
Less developed regions	1,709	4,719	7,754
Africa	221	749	1,766
Asia	1,402	3,585	5,268
Europe	547	729	628
Latin America and the Caribbean	167	504	809
Northern America	172	305	392
Oceania	13	30	46

BACKGROUND AND INTRODUCTION

The three primary drivers leading to increases in the world's vehicle fleets are population growth, increased urbanization and economic improvement. All three trends are up, especially in developing countries.

The global population increased from approximately 2.5 billion people in 1950 to 6 billion in 2002, and it is projected to increase by an additional 50 per cent to 9 billion by 2050. As illustrated in Table 8.1 this growth will not be evenly distributed but will be concentrated outside of the Organisation for Economic Co-operation and Development (OECD), in Asia, Africa and Latin America.

Simultaneously, all regions of the world continue to urbanize (Table 8.2) with the highest rate of urbanization expected in Asia. This is significant since per capita vehicle populations are greater in urban than in rural areas.

According to Peter Wiederker at the OECD, annual gross domestic product (GDP) growth rates over the next two decades will be highest in China, East Asia, Central and Eastern Europe and the former Soviet Union, which will stimulate growth in vehicle populations in these regions (Table 8.3).

Table 8.2 *Proportion of the population living in urban areas and rate of urbanization by major area – 1950, 2000 and 2030*

Major area	Percentage urban			Rate of urbanization (percentage)	
	1950	2000	2030	1950–2000	2000–2030
World	29.8	47.2	60.2	0.92	0.81
Africa	14.7	37.2	52.9	1.86	1.17
Asia	17.4	37.5	54.1	1.53	1.23
Europe	52.4	73.4	80.5	0.68	0.31
Latin America and the Caribbean	41.9	75.4	84.0	1.18	0.36
Northern America	63.9	77.4	84.5	0.38	0.30
Oceania	61.6	74.1	77.3	0.37	0.14

Source: United Nations, 2002

Table 8.3 *The projected annual growth rates in gross domestic product for the regions of the world, %*

Region	1995–2000	2000–2005	2005–2010	2010–2015	2015–2020
Canada, Mexico and United States	2.9	2.5	2.0	1.6	1.6
Western Europe	2.4	2.6	1.5	1.2	1.2
Central and Eastern Europe	3.6	4.5	4.1	3.6	3.6
Japan and Korea	0.75	2.25	1.5	1.0	1.0
Australia and New Zealand	3.0	3.1	2.2	1.75	1.75
Former Soviet Union	−2.5	3.5	4.5	4.0	4.0
China	7.6	5.6	5.0	4.8	4.8
East Asia	2.4	4.8	4.8	4.5	4.2
Latin America	1.75	3.1	2.9	2.8	2.8
Rest of the World	2.75	3.2	3.0	3.0	3.0

As a result of these factors, one can anticipate steady and substantial growth in the global vehicle population. This will be discussed in the next section.

Vehicle Population Trends and Characteristics

Trends in world motor vehicle production

Overall, growth in the production of motor vehicles, especially since the end of World War II, has been quite dramatic, rising from approximately 5 million motor vehicles per year to about 55 million. Between 1950 and now, approximately 1 million additional vehicles have been produced each year (Figure 8.1).

Over the past several decades, motor vehicle production has gradually expanded from one region of the world to another. Initially and through the 1950s, it was dominated by North America. The first wave of competition came from Europe, and by the late 1960s European production had surpassed that of

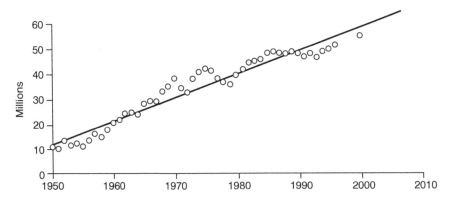

Figure 8.1 *Global trends in motor vehicle (cars, trucks, buses) production*

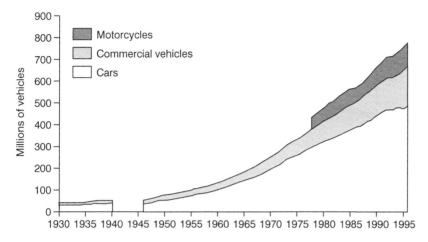

Figure 8.2 *Global trends in motor vehicles*

the US. Between 1980 and 2000 the car industry in Asia, led by Japan, has grown rapidly and now rivals those in the US and Europe. Both Latin America and Eastern Europe appear poised to grow substantially in future decades. For example, driven in large part by Brazil, motor vehicle production in South America now exceeds 2 million units per year.

Motorcycle production has also grown rapidly, especially in Asia. China alone now produces over 10 million motorcycles per year, approximately 50 per cent of the world's total.

Vehicle registrations

Over the past 50 years, the world's vehicle population has grown 15-fold (Figure 8.2). As a result, the global motor vehicle population in 2000 – including passenger cars, trucks, buses, motorcycles and three-wheeled vehicles (tuk tuks)

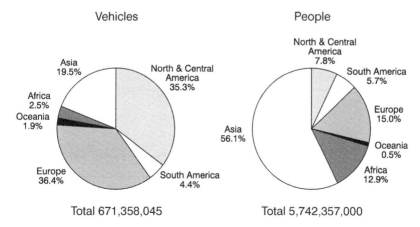

Figure 8.3 *Global distribution of vehicles and people, 1996*

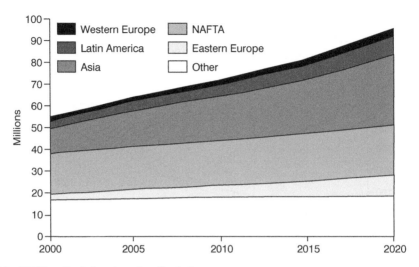

Note: NAFTA = North American Free Trade Area

Figure 8.4 *New vehicle sales forecast (excluding motorcycles)*

– exceeded 700 million units and is projected to reach 1 billion soon.

As illustrated in Figure 8.3, most of these vehicles are concentrated in the highly industrialized countries of the OECD.

However, that is now changing rapidly. As a result, an increasing number of urbanized areas in developing countries are experiencing accelerated growth in vehicle populations and vehicle miles travelled. Nowhere is this more the case than in South-East Asia (Figure 8.4).

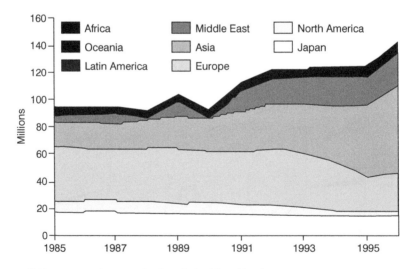

Source: NV Iyer, personal communication, derived from Honda

Figure 8.5 *Motorcycle registrations around the world*

The motorcycle and scooter population is also growing rapidly in Asia (Figure 8.5).

These vehicles have brought many advantages, including increased mobility, economic flexibility, efficiency improvements, more jobs and other quality of life enhancements. However, the benefits have been at least partially offset by excessive pollution and the adverse health and environmental effects that result from air pollution.

ADVERSE HEALTH EFFECTS RESULTING FROM VEHICLE EMISSIONS

Cars, trucks, motorcycles, scooters and buses emit significant quantities of carbon monoxide (CO), hydrocarbons (HCs), nitrogen oxides (NO_x) and fine particles. Where leaded gasoline is used, it is also a significant source of lead in urban air. As a result of the high growth in vehicles and these emissions, many cities in developing countries are severely polluted. The health impacts of these pollutants have been reviewed in Chapters 2 and 3, so this section will review relevant aspects of vehicle emissions and effects on health.

Photochemical oxidants (ozone)

As discussed in the Introduction and Chapter 2, ground-level ozone (O_3), the main ingredient in smog, is formed by complex chemical reactions of volatile organic compounds (VOCs) and NO_x in the presence of heat and sunlight. O_3 forms readily in the lower atmosphere, usually during hot summer weather. VOCs are emitted from a variety of sources, including motor vehicles, chemical plants, refineries, factories, consumer and commercial products and other industrial sources. VOCs also are emitted by natural sources such as vegetation. NO_x is emitted largely from motor vehicles, non-road equipment, power plants and other sources of combustion.

Based on a large number of recent studies, it is clear that serious adverse health effects result when people are exposed to levels of O_3 found today in many areas (see Chapters 2 and 3).

Particulate matter (PM)

PM represents a broad class of chemically and physically diverse substances that exist as discrete particles (liquid droplets or solids) over a wide range of sizes. Human-generated sources of particles include a variety of stationary and mobile sources. Particles may be emitted directly to the atmosphere or may be formed by transformations of gaseous emissions such as sulphur dioxide (SO_2) or NO_x. The major chemical and physical properties of PM vary greatly with the time, region, meteorology and source category, thus complicating the assessment of health and welfare effects as related to various indicators of particulate pollution. At elevated concentrations, PM can adversely affect human health, visibility and materials.

The key health effects categories associated with PM include: premature death; aggravation of respiratory and cardiovascular disease, as indicated by increased hospital admissions and emergency room visits, school absences, work loss days and restricted activity days; changes in lung function and increased respiratory symptoms; changes to lung tissues and structure; and altered respiratory defence mechanisms. Most of these effects have been consistently associated with ambient PM concentrations, which have been used as a measure of population exposure in a large number of community epidemiological studies. Additional information and insights on these effects are provided by studies of animal toxicology and controlled human exposures to various constituents of PM conducted at higher than ambient concentrations. Although the mechanisms by which particles cause effects are not well known, there is general agreement that the cardiorespiratory system is the major target of PM effects.

Individuals with respiratory disease (eg chronic obstructive pulmonary disease or acute bronchitis) and cardiovascular disease (eg ischemic heart disease) are at greater risk of premature mortality and hospitalization due to exposure to ambient PM.

Individuals with infectious respiratory disease (eg pneumonia) are at greater risk of premature mortality and morbidity (eg hospitalization or aggravation of respiratory symptoms) due to exposure to ambient PM. Also, exposure to PM may increase individuals' susceptibility to respiratory infections. Elderly individuals are also at greater risk of premature mortality and hospitalization for cardiopulmonary problems due to exposure to ambient PM. Children are at greater risk of increased respiratory symptoms and decreased lung function due to exposure to ambient PM. Asthmatic individuals are at risk of exacerbation of symptoms associated with asthma and increased need for medical attention due to exposure to PM.

There are fundamental physical and chemical differences between fine and coarse fraction particles. The fine fraction contains acid aerosols, sulphates, nitrates, transition metals, diesel exhaust particles and ultrafine particles, and the coarse fraction typically contains high mineral concentrations, silica and resuspended dust. Exposure to coarse fraction particles is primarily associated with the aggravation of respiratory conditions such as asthma. Fine particles are most closely associated with health effects such as premature death or hospital admissions, and for cardiopulmonary diseases.

Diesel health assessment

Diesel emissions deserve a special discussion because they tend to be a dominant source of mobile-source cancer risk. The US Environmental Protection Agency (EPA) determined a reference concentration in 1993 to minimize non-cancer health effects resulting from exposure to diesel exhaust. The EPA has summarized available information to characterize the cancer and non-cancer health effects from exposure to diesel exhaust emissions in the draft *Health Assessment Document for Diesel Emissions*. The key components of the Assessment are:

- information about the chemical components of diesel exhaust and how they can influence toxicity,
- the cancer and non-cancer health effects of concern for humans, and
- the possible impact or risk to an exposed human population.

The US EPA has concluded that diesel particulate is a probable human carcinogen. The most compelling information to suggest a carcinogenic hazard is the consistent association that has been observed between increased lung cancer and diesel exhaust exposure in certain occupationally exposed workers working in the presence of diesel engines (National Institute for Occupational Safety and Health, 1988; Health Effects Institute, 1995; World Health Organization, 1996). Approximately 30 individual epidemiological studies show increased lung cancer risks of 20 to 89 per cent within the study populations, depending on the study. The analytical results of pooling the positive study results show that on average the lung cancer risks were increased by 33 to 47 per cent. The magnitude of the pooled risk increases is not precise owing to uncertainties in the individual studies, the most important of which is a continuing concern about whether smoking effects have been accounted for adequately. While not all studies have demonstrated an increased risk (6 of 34 epidemiological studies reported relative risks less than 1 (Health Effects Institute, 1995)), the fact that an increased risk has been consistently noted in the majority of epidemiological studies strongly supports the determination that exposure to diesel exhaust is likely to pose a carcinogenic hazard to humans.

Additional evidence for treating diesel exhaust as a carcinogen at ambient levels of exposure is provided by the observation of the presence of small quantities of many mutagenic and some carcinogenic compounds in the diesel exhaust. A carcinogenic response believed to be caused by such agents is assumed not to have a threshold unless there is direct evidence to the contrary. In addition, there is evidence that at least some of the organic compounds associated with diesel PM are extracted by lung fluids (ie, are bio-available) and, therefore, are available in some quantity to the lungs as well as entering the bloodstream and being transported to other sites in the body.

The concern for the carcinogenic health hazard resulting from diesel exhaust exposures is widespread, and several national and international agencies have designated diesel exhaust or diesel PM as a 'potential' or 'probable' human carcinogen (National Institute for Occupational Safety and Health, 1988; World Health Organization, 1996). The International Agency for Research on Cancer (IARC) concluded that diesel exhaust is a 'probable' human carcinogen (IARC, 1989). Based on IARC findings, in 1990 California identified diesel exhaust as a chemical known to cause cancer and after an extensive review in 1998 listed diesel exhaust as a toxic air contaminant (California EPA, 1998). The World Health Organization recommends that 'urgent efforts should be made to reduce [diesel engine] emissions, specifically of particulates, by changing exhaust train techniques, engine design and fuel composition' (World Health Organization, 1996).

Another aspect of diesel particulate that is a cause for concern is its size. Approximately 80–95 per cent of diesel particle mass is in the size range from

0.05–1 microns with a mean particle diameter of about 0.2 microns. These fine particles have a very large surface area per gram of mass, which make them excellent carriers for adsorbed inorganic and organic compounds that can effectively reach the lowest airways of the lung. Approximately 50–90 per cent of the number of particles in diesel exhaust are in the ultrafine size range from 0.005–0.05 microns, averaging about 0.02 microns. While accounting for the majority of the number of particles, ultrafine diesel PM accounts for 1–20 per cent of the mass of diesel PM.

The MATES study

The Multiple Air Toxics Exposure Study (MATES-II) is a landmark urban toxics monitoring and evaluation study conducted for the South Coast Air Basin. It represents one of the most comprehensive air toxics programmes ever conducted in an urban environment. It consists of several elements: a comprehensive monitoring programme, an updated emissions inventory of toxic air contaminants and a modelling effort to fully characterize Basin risk.

In the monitoring programme, over 30 air pollutants were measured, including both gas and particulates (Table 8.4).

When 'carcinogenic risk' is discussed, it typically refers to the probability of a person contracting cancer over the course of a lifetime if exposed to the source of cancer-causing compounds for 70 years. In other words, a cancer risk of 100 in a million at a location means that individuals staying at that location for 70 years have a 100 in a million chance of contracting cancer. If 10,000 people live at that location, then the cancer burden for this population will be one (the population multiplied by the cancer risk). This means that one of the 10,000 people staying at the location for 70 years is expected to contract cancer.

Table 8.4 *Pollutants measured in MATES-II*

Chemical name	Chemical name
Benzene	Formaldehyde
1,3-Butadiene	Acetaldehyde
Dichlorobenzene (ortho- and para)	Acetone
Vinyl chloride	Arsenic
Ethyl benzene	Chromium
Toluene	Lead
Xylene (m-, p-, o-)	Nickel
Styrene	Cobalt
Carbon tetrachloride	Copper
Chloroform	Manganese
Dichloroethane [1,1]	Phosphorus
Dichloroethylene [1,1]	Selenium
Methylene chloride	Silica
Perchloroethylene	Silver
Trichloroethylene	Zinc
Chloromethane	PAHs
Organic carbon	Elemental carbon

Source: www.aqmd.gov/news1/MATES_II_results.htm

The key result of the MATES-II study was that the average carcinogenic risk in the Basin is about 1400 per million people. Mobile sources (eg cars, trucks, trains, ships, aircraft etc) represent the greatest contributors. About 70 per cent of all risk is attributed to diesel particulate emissions; about 20 per cent is attributed to other toxics associated with mobile sources (including benzene, butadiene and formaldehyde); and about 10 per cent of all risk is attributed to stationary sources (which include industries and certain other businesses such as dry cleaners and chrome plating operations).

The carcinogenic risk of 1400 per million is based on a range from approximately 1120 in a million to approximately 1740 in a million among the ten sites.

Nitrogen oxides (NO$_x$)

As a class of compounds, the oxides of nitrogen are involved in a host of environmental concerns impacting adversely on human health and welfare. Nitrogen dioxide (NO$_2$) has been linked with increased susceptibility to respiratory infection, increased airway resistance in asthmatics and decreased pulmonary function (US EPA, 1993, 1995). NO$_x$ is a principal cause of O$_3$ formation as noted earlier. NO$_x$ also is a contributor to acid deposition, which can damage trees at high elevations and increases the acidity of lakes and streams, which can severely damage aquatic life. Finally, NO$_x$ emissions can contribute to increased levels of PM by changing into nitric acid in the atmosphere and forming particulate nitrate, as also noted earlier.

Carbon monoxide (CO)

CO – an odourless, invisible gas created when fuels containing carbon are burned incompletely – poses a serious threat to human health, as discussed in Chapters 2 and 3. Persons afflicted with heart disease and foetuses are especially at risk. Because the affinity of haemoglobin in the blood is 200 times greater for CO than for oxygen, CO hinders oxygen transport from blood into tissues. Therefore, more blood must be pumped to deliver the same amount of oxygen. Numerous studies in humans and animals have demonstrated that those individuals with weak hearts are placed under additional strain by the presence of excess CO in the blood. In particular, clinical health studies have shown a decrease in time to onset of angina pain in those individuals suffering from angina pectoris and exposed to elevated levels of ambient CO.

Healthy individuals also are affected, but only at higher levels. Exposure to elevated CO levels is associated with impairment of visual perception, work capacity, manual dexterity, learning ability and performance of complex tasks (US EPA, 1999).

Other air toxics from engines and vehicles

In addition to contributing to the health and welfare problems associated with exceedances of the air quality standards for O$_3$ and PM$_{10}$, emissions from diesel and gasoline vehicles include a number of air pollutants that increase the risk of cancer or have other negative health effects. These air pollutants include benzene, formaldehyde, acetaldehyde, 1,3-butadiene and diesel PM (discussed earlier). All of these compounds are products of combustion; benzene is also found in non-exhaust emissions from gasoline-fuelled vehicles.

There are hundreds of different compounds and elements that are known to be emitted from passenger cars, on-highway trucks and various pieces of non-road equipment. The US EPA (1999) has proposed a methodology for identifying which of these compounds and elements are toxic, and has developed a preliminary mobile source air toxics (MSAT) list.

The methodology uses the Integrated Risk Information System (IRIS), which is a US EPA database of scientific information that contains the Agency consensus scientific positions on potential adverse health effects that may result from lifetime (chronic) or short term (acute) exposure to various substances found in the environment. IRIS currently provides health effects information on over 500 specific chemical compounds. The information contained in the IRIS database includes an EPA finding for each compound that:

- there is a health hazard, either cancer or non-cancer, associated with exposure to the compound;
- the compound is non-carcinogenic based on current data; or
- the data is insufficient to determine whether the compound is a hazard.

IRIS contains chemical-specific summaries of qualitative and quantitative health information. IRIS information may include the reference dose (RfD) for non-cancer health effects resulting from oral exposure, the reference concentration (RfC) for non-cancer health effects resulting from inhalation exposure, and the carcinogen assessment for both oral and inhalation exposure. Combined with information on specific exposure situations, the summary health hazard information in IRIS may be used in evaluating potential public health risks from environmental contaminants.

By comparing the list of compounds in IRIS to the motor vehicle emissions identified in the speciation studies, EPA identified 21 MSATs as listed in Table 8.5. Each of these pollutants is a known, probable or possible human carcinogen (Group A, B or C) or is considered by the US EPA to pose a risk of adverse non-cancer health effects.

Gaseous air toxics

Benzene

Benzene is an aromatic HC that is present as a gas in both exhaust and evaporative emissions from motor vehicles. Benzene in the exhaust, expressed as a percentage of total organic gases (TOG), varies depending on the control technology (eg type of catalyst) and the levels of benzene and other aromatics in the fuel, but is generally about 3–5 per cent. The benzene fraction of evaporative emissions depends on control technology and fuel composition and characteristics (eg benzene level and the evaporation rate) and is generally about 1 per cent (US EPA, 1999).

Table 8.5 *Proposed list of mobile source air toxics*

Acetaldehyde	Diesel exhaust	MTBE***
Acrolein	Ethylbenzene	Naphthalene
Arsenic compounds*	Formaldehyde	Nickel compounds*
Benzene	n–Hexane	POM****
1,3-Butadiene	Lead compounds*	Styrene
Chromium compounds*	Manganese compounds*	Toluene
Dioxin/furans**	Mercury compounds*	Xylene

Notes: * = Although the different species of the same metal differ in their toxicity, the on-road mobile source inventory contains emissions estimates for total compounds of the metal identified in particulate speciation profiles (ie, the sum of all forms).
** = This entry refers to two large groups of chlorinated compounds. In assessing their cancer risks, their quantitative potencies are usually derived from that of the most toxic, 2,3,7,8-tetrachlorodibenzodioxin.
*** = MTBE is listed due to its potential inhalation air toxics effects and not due to ingestion exposure associated with drinking water contamination.
**** = Polycyclic organic matter (POM) includes organic compounds with more than one benzene ring, and which have a boiling point greater than or equal to 100 degrees centigrade. A group of seven polynuclear aromatic hydrocarbons, which have been identified by EPA as probable human carcinogens (benz(a)anthracene, benzo(b)fluoranthene, benzo(k)fluoranthene, benzo(a)pyrene, chrysene, 7,12-dimethylbenz(a)anthracene and indeno(1,2,3-cd)pyrene) are sometimes used as a surrogate for the larger group of POM compounds.

The EPA has recently reconfirmed that benzene is a known human carcinogen by all routes of exposure (US EPA, 1998). The World Health Organization considers benzene to be carcinogenic to humans and no safe level of exposure can be recommended (WHO, 2000). Respiration is the major source of human exposure. Long term respiratory exposure to high levels of ambient benzene concentrations has been shown to cause cancer of the tissues that form white blood cells.

A number of adverse non-cancer health effects, including blood disorders such as pre-leukemia and aplastic anaemia, have also been associated with low dose, long term exposure to benzene (Lumley, Barker and Murray, 1990). People with long term exposure to benzene may experience harmful effects on the blood-forming tissues, especially the bone marrow. These effects can disrupt normal blood production and cause a decrease in important blood components, such as red blood cells and blood platelets, leading to anaemia (a reduction in the number of red blood cells), leukopenia (a reduction in the number of white blood cells) or thrombocytopenia (a reduction in the number of blood platelets, thus reducing the ability of blood to clot).

Formaldehyde

Formaldehyde is the most prevalent aldehyde in vehicle exhaust. It is formed from incomplete combustion of both gasoline and diesel fuel and accounts for 1–4 per cent of total exhaust TOG emissions, depending on control technology and fuel composition. It is not found in evaporative emissions.

Formaldehyde exhibits extremely complex atmospheric behaviour (US EPA, 1993). It is formed by the atmospheric oxidation of virtually all organic species, including biogenic (produced by a living organism) HCs. Mobile sources contribute both primary formaldehyde (emitted directly from motor vehicles) and secondary formaldehyde (formed from photo-oxidation of other VOCs emitted from vehicles).

The US EPA has classified formaldehyde as a probable human carcinogen based on limited evidence for carcinogenicity in humans and sufficient evidence of carcinogenicity in animal studies, rats, mice, hamsters and monkeys (US EPA, 1993). The IARC considers that there is limited evidence that formaldehyde is carcinogenic to humans (category 2A) (IARC, 1995). Epidemiological studies in occupationally exposed workers suggest that the long term inhalation of formaldehyde may be associated with tumours of the nasopharyngeal cavity (generally the area at the back of the mouth near the nose), the nasal cavity and the sinus. Studies in experimental animals provide sufficient evidence that long term inhalation exposure to formaldehyde causes an increase in the incidence of squamous (epithelial) cell carcinomas (tumours) of the nasal cavity.

It is estimated that approximately one person in one million exposed to 1 milligram per cubic metre (mg/m^3) of formaldehyde continuously for their lifetime (70 years) would develop cancer as a result of this exposure.

Formaldehyde exposure also causes a range of non-cancer health effects. At low concentrations (0.05–2.0 parts per million, ppm), irritation of the eyes (tearing of the eyes and increased blinking) and mucous membranes is the principal effect observed in humans. At exposure to 1–11ppm, other human upper respiratory effects associated with acute formaldehyde exposure include a dry or sore throat and a tingling sensation of the nose. Sensitive individuals may experience these effects at lower concentrations.

Acetaldehyde

Acetaldehyde is a saturated aldehyde that is found in vehicle exhaust and is formed as a result of incomplete combustion of both gasoline and diesel fuel. It is not a component of evaporative emissions. Acetaldehyde comprises 0.4–1 per cent of exhaust TOG, depending on control technology and fuel composition (US EPA, 1999).

The atmospheric chemistry of acetaldehyde is similar in many respects to that of formaldehyde. Like formaldehyde, it is produced and destroyed by atmospheric chemical transformation. Mobile sources contribute to ambient acetaldehyde levels both by their primary emissions and by secondary formation resulting from their VOC emissions. Acetaldehyde emissions are classified by the US EPA as a Group B2 probable human carcinogen. It is estimated that less than one person in one million exposed to $1mg/m^3$ acetaldehyde continuously for their lifetime (70 years) would develop cancer as a result of their exposure.

Non-cancer effects in studies with rats and mice showed acetaldehyde to be moderately toxic by the inhalation, oral and intravenous routes (US EPA, 1987). The primary acute effect of exposure to acetaldehyde vapours is irritation of the eyes, skin and respiratory tract. At high concentrations, irritation and pulmonary effects can occur, which could facilitate the uptake of other contaminants. Little research exists that addresses the effects of inhalation of acetaldehyde on reproductive and developmental effects. The in vitro and in vivo studies provide evidence to suggest that acetaldehyde may be the causative factor in birth defects observed in foetal alcohol syndrome, though evidence is very limited linking these effects to inhalation exposure. Long term exposures should be kept below the reference concentration of $9mg/m^3$ to avoid appreciable risk of these non-cancer health effects (US EPA, 1999).

1,3–Butadiene

1,3–Butadiene is formed in vehicle exhaust by the incomplete combustion of fuel. It is not present in vehicle evaporative emissions, because it is not present in any appreciable amount in fuel. 1,3–Butadiene accounts for 0.4 to 1 per cent of total exhaust TOG, depending on control technology and fuel composition (US EPA, 1999).

   1,3–Butadiene is classified by the EPA as a Group B2 (probable human carcinogen) (US EPA, 1985). The IARC classified 1,3-butadiene as probably carcinogenic to humans (category 2A) (WHO, 2000). It is estimated that approximately two people in one million exposed to $1\mu g/m^3$ 1,3-butadiene continuously for their lifetime (70 years) would develop cancer as a result of their exposure (US EPA, 1999).

   An adjustment factor of three can be applied to this potency estimate to reflect evidence from rodent studies suggesting that extrapolating the excess risk of leukaemia in a male-only occupational cohort may underestimate the total cancer risk from 1,3-butadiene exposure in the general population.

   Long term exposures to 1,3-butadiene should be kept below its reference concentration of $4\mu g/m^3$ to avoid appreciable risks of these reproductive and developmental effects (US EPA, 1985).

Acrolein

Acrolein is extremely toxic to humans from the inhalation route of exposure, with acute exposure resulting in upper respiratory tract irritation and congestion. The US EPA RfC for inhalation of acrolein is $0.02\mu g/m^3$. Although no information is available on its carcinogenic effects in humans, based on laboratory animal data the US EPA considers acrolein a possible human carcinogen (US EPA, 1993).

STRATEGIES TO REDUCE VEHICLE EMISSIONS

Reducing the pollution that comes from vehicles will usually require a comprehensive strategy as shown below. Generally, the goal of a motor vehicle pollution control programme is to reduce emissions from the motor vehicles in use to the degree reasonably necessary to achieve healthy air quality as rapidly as possible or, failing that for reasons of impracticality, to the practical limits of effective technological, economic and social feasibility. A comprehensive strategy to achieve this goal includes four key components: stringent emissions standards for new vehicles, clean fuels, programmes to assure proper

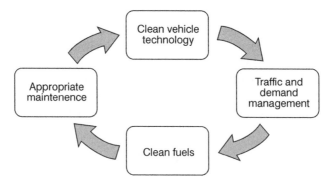

Figure 8.6 *Elements of a comprehensive vehicle pollution control strategy*

maintenance of in-use vehicles, and traffic and demand management (Figure 8.6). The emission reduction goal should be achieved in the most cost-effective manner available.

Throughout the developing world, air pollution is a serious problem. Cities as diverse as Hong Kong, Delhi, Bangkok, Sao Paulo and Seoul, to cite just a few, currently exceed healthy air quality levels, sometimes by a factor of two or three. In Taipei for example, PM_{10} and O_3 air quality standards are exceeded several times per year. In Bangkok, it is estimated that roadside emissions of PM, CO and lead must be reduced by 85 per cent, 47 per cent and 13 per cent respectively if acceptable air quality is to be achieved.

While many sources contribute to pollution in these cities, vehicles clearly stand out as major sources. Vehicles emit approximately 80 per cent of the CO in both Beijing and Guangzhou in China and almost 40 per cent of the NO_x; in Delhi, vehicles are the major source of HCs, NO_x and carbon dioxide (CO_2).

In heavy traffic areas of Hong Kong, diesel vehicles have been found to be responsible for more than half the respirable particles; at two locations in Bangkok motorcycles were found to be the major source of particulate air pollution.

Control efforts in Taiwan

A few years ago, the Taiwan EPA took advantage of routine air raid drills in three major urban areas – Taipei, Taichung and Kaohsiung – to determine the impact of vehicles. During air raids, all traffic is required to stop and vehicle engines are turned off. By comparing air quality readings before and during the drills, the role of motor vehicles can be ascertained. The results summarized in Table 8.6 indicate that CO and NO_x concentrations fell by about 80 per cent after vehicles came to a halt, and that levels quickly returned to normal once traffic began moving.

The survey results clearly indicate the substantial degree to which motor vehicles contribute to air pollution in urban areas. Serious pollution problems, however, are not inevitable. For example, in Taiwan the emission standard for third stage of automobiles, third stage of motorcycles and third stage of diesel

Table 8.6 *Comparison of air pollution in urban areas between traffic and non-traffic situations*

Pollutant	Taipei		Taichung	Kaohsiung
CO	Average concentration (ppm)	3.00	1.50	3.00
	Vehicles stationary (ppm)	0.50	0.50	0.50
	Reduction (%)	83.33	66.67	83.33
NO_x	Average concentration (ppb)	300.00	60.00	200.00
	Vehicles stationary (ppb)	50.00	10.00	50.00
	Reduction (%)	83.33	83.33	75.00

vehicles went into effect on January 1 1999, January 1 1998 and July 1 1999 respectively (Tables 8.7 and 8.8).

Following numerous discussions with industry, the Taiwan EPA completed a draft version of motorcycle emission control standards. In addition to tightening emission limits, these standards regulate two- and four-stroke motorcycle models separately and require cold-engine emissions testing. The new standards will tighten limits on CO, HCs and NO_x by as much as 80 per cent (see Table 8.9).

The Taiwan EPA announced on August 5 1999 that these standards are to go into effect on January 1 2004. Firms closely watching the development of the fourth stage standards dubbed them the 'terminating' articles for two-stroke motorcycles. The following is a list of the main features of the fourth stage standards:

1 They set different emission standards for two- and four-stroke motorcycles. First, second and third stage standards used the same standards for both

Table 8.7 *The emission standards for automobiles in Taiwan (Taiwan EPA)*

Vehicle	Weight	Effective date	CO (g/km)	HC (g/km)	NO_x (g/km)	PM (g/km)
Gasoline	<3.5t	1/7/90	2.11	0.255	0.62	–
passenger		1/1/99	2.11	0.155	0.25	
vehicles						
Gasoline	<1200cc	1/7/95	11.18	1.06	1.43	–
goods	<1200cc	1/1/99	6.20	0.50	1.43	–
vehicles &	>1200cc	1/7/95	6.20	0.50	1.43	–
buses	>1200cc	1/1/99	3.11	0.242	0.68	–
Light duty	GVW<2.5t	1/7/93	6.2	0.5	1.4	0.38
diesel		1/7/98	2.125	0.156	0.25	0.05
			g/bhp-hr	g/bhp-hr	g/bhp-hr	g/bhp-hr
Heavy duty	GVW>3.5t	1/7/93	10.0	1.3	6.0	0.7
diesel	1/7/99		10.0	1.3	5.0	0.1

Note: t = tonnes; cc = cubic centimetres equivalent to millilitres; g/km = grams per kilometre; g/bhp-hr = grams per brake horsepower-hour.

Table 8.8 *The emission standards for motorcycles in Taiwan (Taiwan EPA)*

Year	Test	Durability (km)	CO (g/km)	HC + NO$_x$ (g/km)
1988	ECE R40	–	8.8	5.5
1991	ECE R40	6000	4.5	3.0
1998	ECE R40	15,000	3.5	2.0

two- and four-stroke motorcycles. According to investigation results, however, the average emissions value of a cold-engine-tested two-stroke motorcycle was about triple that of a four-stroke motorcycle and the results were even worse when the motorcycle was in poor condition. For this reason, the standards for two-stroke motorcycles in the fourth stage standards are twice as strict as those for four-stroke motorcycles.

2   They change the tests from warm to cold engine. First, second and third stage standards testing procedures all used the warm engine method, whereby tests were conducted after the motorcycle was driven for 10km until the engine was warm. According to the EPA, investigations indicated that about 70 per cent of trips averaged less than 10km for a round trip, with a one-way journey of no more than 5km. Moreover, the actual quantity of emissions detected in a cold engine test was 2.5 times that of a warm engine test.

3   They tighten emission standards for in-use motorcycles. For the sake of convenience, the standards for CO and HC used to audit in-use motorcycles remained for many years at an average of 4.5 per cent and 9000ppm respectively. Given the increased performance of motorcycles and to ensure that catalytic converters continue to be used, these are to be tightened to 3.5 per cent and 2000ppm respectively. In the future, in-use motorcycles that are not properly maintained may have trouble passing inspection.

Table 8.9 *Current and proposed emission limits for motorcycles*[*]

Engine testing condition	Pollutant	Current (Third stage) 2-, 4-stroke (warm test)	January 1 2004 2-stroke (cold test)	January 1 2004 4-stroke (cold test)
New	Driving cycle test	CO (g/km)	3.5	7.0	7.0
		HC + NO$_x$ (g/km)	2.0	1.0	2.0
	Idle test	CO (%)	4.0	3.0	3.0
		HC (ppm)	6000	2000	2000
In use	Idle	CO (%)	4.5	3.5[**]	3.5[**]
		HC (ppm)	9000	2000[**]	2000[**]

Notes: Average cold engine tested values of CO and HC + NO$_x$ were 2.5 times those of warm engine tested values.
* = Includes scooters and mopeds.
** = Limits for warm engine test conditions.

Two-stroke models currently account for about half of all motorcycles. Under current conditions, two-stroke models are likely to have trouble adjusting to the fourth stage standards when they go into effect and thus two-stroke motorcycles are likely to be eliminated.

In terms of emissions from moving motorcycles, rough estimates indicate that two- and four-stroke emissions improvement rates for CO are to average 20 per cent, and HC + NO_x are to be 80 per cent and 60 per cent, respectively. Assuming each motorcycle ride averages 10km per round trip and 300 rides per year, annual emission reductions of CO and HC + NO_x would be 6000 and 10,000 metric tons respectively.

For idling motorcycles, improvement rates for CO and HC are to be 25 per cent and 67 per cent respectively, which should reduce the concentration of waste gases appreciably during traffic hours and at major intersections in urban areas.

Singapore's land transport policy

Singapore's land transport policy strives to provide free-flowing traffic within the constraint of limited land. A four-pronged approach has been adopted to achieve this. First, the need to travel is minimized through systematic town planning. Second, an extensive and comprehensive network of roads and expressways, augmented by traffic management measures, has been built to provide quick accessibility to all parts of Singapore. Third, a viable and efficient public transport system that integrates both the mass rapid transit (MRT) and bus services is promoted. Finally, the growth and use of vehicles are managed to prevent congestion on the road.

China making progress

One result of the rapid growth in the vehicle population to date in China has been a significant increase in urban air pollution. In spite of significant advances in industrial pollution control, air pollution in the major Chinese cities remains a serious problem and in some cases may actually be worsening. It is generally characterized as a shift from coal-based pollution to vehicle-based pollution.

Based on the available data, it is clear that national NO_x air quality standards are currently exceeded across large areas in China, including but not limited to high traffic areas. Before 1992, the annual average concentration of NO_x in Shanghai was lower than $0.05mg/m^3$, which complies with China's Class II air quality standard. But since 1995, the NO_x concentration has been gradually increasing, from $0.051mg/m^3$ in 1995 to $0.059mg/m^3$ in 1997 (Shanghai Municipal Government, 1999).

In Beijing, NO_x concentrations within the second ring road that encircles the city centre increased from $99mg/m^3$ in 1986 to $205mg/m^3$ in 1997, more than doubling in a decade. Moreover, CO and NO_x concentrations on the urban trunk traffic roads and interchanges exceed national environmental quality standards all year round (Beijing Municipal Environment Protection Bureau, 1999). National air quality standards for particulates are also frequently exceeded, primarily due to coal and charcoal burning.

Table 8.10 O_3 *concentration in Beijing*

	Number of non-attainment days	Number of non-attainment hours	Maximum hourly concentration ($\mu g/m^3$)
1997	71	434	346
1998	101	504	384
1999	119	777	

Recent data also indicate that standards for O_3 have been exceeded in several metropolitan areas during the last decade. For example, Table 8.10 shows a clear upwards trend in Beijing.

On average, mobile sources are currently contributing approximately 45–60 per cent of the NO_x emissions and about 85 per cent of the CO emissions in typical Chinese cities. Recent data collected in Shanghai, for example, show that in 1996, vehicles emitted 86 per cent of the CO, 56 per cent of the NO_x and 96 per cent of the non-methane HCs of the total air pollution load in the downtown area (Shanghai Municipal Government, 1999). In Beijing in recent years, the NO_x concentration shows a clear increasing trend. Annual average NO_x concentrations, average concentrations during the heating season and those during the non-heating season in 1997 were $133\mu g/m^3$, $191\mu g/m^3$ and $99\mu g/m^3$, respectively. These emissions were 73 per cent, 66 per cent and 80 per cent higher than those ten years ago. The annual daily average NO_x concentration in 1998 was 14.3 per cent higher than in 1997. Since the amount of coal burning has remained stable for many years, Beijing local authorities attribute the increases to vehicular emissions (Beijing Municipal Environment Protection Bureau, 1999). As noted by the Beijing EPB:

> *in 2000, NO_x emissions by motor vehicles accounted for 43 per cent of the total and CO emission, 83 per cent. As the vehicles discharge pollutants at low altitude, they contribute to 73 per cent and 84 per cent of the effect on environmental quality.* (Yu Xiaoxuan, Beijing Environmental Protection Bureau.)

To deal with the problems of air pollution, China has initiated a significant motor vehicle pollution control effort. It has moved quickly to eliminate the use of leaded gasoline and recently introduced EURO 1 standards for new cars and trucks. It has also been decided to introduce the EURO 2 standards in 2004. However, in spite of this, the emissions requirements for new vehicles lag behind those of the industrialized world by approximately a decade. Further, without additional fuel quality improvements, the additional tightening of new vehicle standards will be difficult. In addition, road conditions and maintenance practices are considered to be causing higher in-use emissions compared with comparable cars in the industrialized countries.

Table 8.11 *Percentage violation of National Ambient Air Quality Standards in Delhi*

Parameter	1995	1996	1997	1998	1999
Sulphur dioxide[*]	7.0%	2.4%	0.4%	0.0%	0.0%
Nitrogen dioxide[*]	21.0%	35.5%	21.8%	20.7%	14.8%
Suspended particulate matter[*]	95.1%	97.2%	98.4%	97.0%	96.0%
Respirable particulate matter (PM_{10})[*]	–	–	89.0%	88.0%	86.7%
Carbon monoxide[**]	70.8%	86.0%	94.3%	86.3%	87.4%

Notes: [*] = based on a 245-hour standard.
[**] = based on an 8-hour standard.

Recent progress in India

Air pollution levels in India are very poor, among the worst in the world for particulate as indicated in Tables 8.11 and 8.12. Levels of suspended particulate exceed India's air quality standards on almost every day of the year and usually by multiple factors. Further, high levels of particulate are not limited to one city or region but appear to be widely distributed all across the country.

Vehicle population

The vehicle fleet in the country as a whole as well as in the capital, Delhi, is dominated by two-wheeled vehicles, as shown below (Table 8.13).

New vehicle standards

Standards for all categories of vehicles have been gradually tightened over the past decade but especially within the past few years.

Table 8.12 *Annual average concentration of particulate in various cities in India ($\mu g/m^3$)*

State	City	PM_{10}	SPM	% PM_{10} in SPM
Gujarat	Ahmedabad (R)	165	312	53
Andra Pradesh	Hyderabad (R)	106	223	48
	Hyderabad (I)	164	370	44
	Vishakhapatnam (R)	74	193	38
	Vishakapatnam (I)	69	145	48
Tamil Nadu	Chennai (R)	75	77	97
Uttar Pradesh	Kanpur (R)	342	337	72
	Dehradun (R)	152	340	45
Delhi	Delhi (R)	206	351	59
	Delhi (traffic intersection)	216	418	52
Maharashtra	Mumbai (R)	115	247	47
West Bengal	Calcutta (R)	138	268	52
NAAQS	Industrial area	120	360	
	Residential area	60	140	

Note: R = residential area; I = industrial area.

Table 8.13 *A summary of existing and planned fuel specifications in India (Ministry of Surface Transport, New Delhi)*

	Metros	TAJ Trapezium region	State capitals	Entire country
Low sulphur diesel				
Up to 0.5%	April 1 1996	April 1 1996		
Up to 0.25%		September 1 1996		September 1 1999
Low lead petrol	June 1	September 1		December 1996
(0.15g/litre)	1994	1995		
Unleaded petrol	April 1	April 1	December 31	March 31
(0.013g/litre)	1995	1995	1998	2000

Fuels requirements

Tighter new vehicle standards have been made possible through the widespread availability of unleaded petrol.

The sulphur levels in diesel fuel remain quite high and will soon become a significant impediment to tighter new vehicle standards.

In-use vehicles

With regard to in-use vehicles, all four-wheeled petrol-fuelled vehicles are required to meet a standard of 3 per cent CO when measured at idle; two- and three-wheeled vehicles must meet a standard of 4.5 per cent CO. With regard to diesel vehicles, all but agricultural tractors must meet a smoke density requirement of no more than 75 Hartridge Smoke Units (HSU) when tested at full load, 70 per cent maximum revolutions per minute (RPM) or 65 HSU when tested by the free acceleration test.

Recent steps to reduce vehicle emissions include the following:

- **Unleaded petrol:** as of September 1998, only unleaded gasoline has been sold in Delhi with the result that there has already been a reduction of lead in the air by more than 60 per cent. Industry has also been asked to ensure that benzene emissions do not increase and to constrain the benzene content in unleaded fuel to 5 per cent, the level proposed for leaded gasoline in 1996. By 2000 the level was reduced to 3 per cent in Delhi only. Leaded petrol was banned throughout the country by April 2000.
- **Other fuel parameters:** the Supreme Court directed the Ministry of Petroleum and Natural Gas to ensure that the region of Delhi (which includes the national capital itself and bordering districts of adjoining states) be supplied with petrol with a maximum sulphur content of 0.05 per cent by 31 May 2000, petrol with a maximum benzene content of 1 per cent by 31 March 2001 and diesel with a maximum sulphur content of 0.05 per cent by 30 June 2001.

- **CNG conversions:** another debate focused on introducing compressed natural gas (CNG) on the existing fleet of buses, since the Supreme Court ordered that all buses more than eight years old were to be run on CNG in Delhi from April 1 2000. From 2001 the entire fleet was expected to run on CNG.
- **Emissions standards for new vehicles:** the national Ministry of Surface Transport has extended the Bharat Stage II emissions standards (equivalent to Euro II) for passenger cars to the other metro cities. It may be recalled that the Euro II equivalent emissions standards for passenger cars were enforced in Delhi under an order of the Supreme Court from April 1 2000. According to the notification, the dates of enforcement were to be January 1 2001 in Mumbai and July 1 2001 in Kolkata and Chennai. The date of enforcement for Mumbai was in keeping with the order of the Mumbai High Court. However, for Kolkata, the Department of Environment of the West Bengal government issued an order bringing the date of implementation of the 'Bharat Stage II' standard forward to November 1 2000. Since the availability of fuels of desired quality was a prerequisite for complying with the new standards, the West Bengal notification confirmed that both petrol and diesel with a maximum sulphur content of 0.05 per cent would be available in Kolkata from November 1 2000.
- **Oil for two-stroke (2T) engines:** pre-mixed oil dispensers have been installed in all the petrol filling stations of Delhi and the sale of loose 2T oil has been banned since December 1998. Further, the Ministry of Environment and Forests has required the use of low smoke 2T oil since April 1 1999.
- **Phase-out of old vehicles:** since December 1998, commercial vehicles older than 15 years have been phased out.

Steps taken to date have begun to reduce pollution in Delhi although, with the exception of ambient lead, the reductions have been very modest. Therefore additional control measures are under discussion, including:

- Improvement of public transport.
- Optimization of traffic flow and improved traffic management.
- Upgraded inspection and maintenance system.
- Phase-out of gross polluters.
- Additional fuel quality improvements including lower benzene and aromatics in gasoline, reformulated gasoline and lower sulphur in diesel fuel.
- Euro 4 standards by 2005.
- Restrictions on two-stroke engines, introduction of onboard diagnostics.
- Stopping fuel adulteration.
- Stage 1 vapour recovery systems.
- SIAM road map (the Society of Indian Automobile Manufacturers (SIAM) has submitted to the government a road map for a progressive reduction in emissions).

- Bharat Stage II-compliant four-wheeled non-commercial vehicles, light commercial vehicles and city buses in nine principal cities within six months of notification if fuel with 0.05 per cent sulphur is made available.
- Passenger cars meeting Euro III equivalent standards from April 1 2004 and Euro IV equivalent standards from 2007. This would be subject to the availability of petrol with a maximum sulphur content of 150ppm and diesel with a maximum sulphur content of 350ppm.
- For commercial vehicles, SIAM has offered to comply with Bharat Stage II standards from April 1 2003 over the whole country, subject to the availability of diesel with 0.05 per cent sulphur. It has proposed to skip the Euro III stage and go directly to Euro IV by 2008 provided that diesel with a maximum of 50ppm sulphur is available.
- For two-wheelers, SIAM has proposed emissions standards of 1.5 grams per kilometre (g/km) for CO and 1.5g/km for HC + NO_x from 2005 (a 25 per cent reduction from the current 2000 standards). It has suggested targets of 1.25g/km for both of the pollutants in 2009 but wants a review of these standards in 2005. Similar levels of reduction are proposed for three-wheelers.
- Alternative fuels. In July 1998, the Supreme Court ordered the replacement of all three-wheeled auto-rickshaws registered in Delhi before 1990 with new ones running on CNG. The auto-rickshaw is a popular form of public transport and is used as a taxi in most Indian cities. Bajaj Auto Ltd, the largest manufacturer of these vehicles in India, launched a new CNG-operated three-wheeled vehicle in Delhi. As of 2000, over 2500 of these vehicles were already on the road and the company expected to replace all the 18,000 pre-1990 vehicles by end of March 2001.

The Indian Motor Vehicles Act prohibits the use of liquefied petroleum gas (LPG) as an automotive fuel. The main reason for this is that it is sold at a subsidized price primarily as a kitchen fuel by the government-controlled oil industry. A few years ago, the LPG sector was opened up to private operators who could import, bottle and sell the gas to industrial and commercial users without any subsidy. Since LPG is considered an environmentally cleaner fuel, the Indian parliament has recently passed a bill seeking to remove any restrictions on use of LPG as an automotive fuel. The government is now expected to issue the necessary notifications and safety standards.

The current situation in Sao Paulo

In spite of vigorous and effective efforts to control emissions from industrial sources, air quality in the Sao Paulo Metropolitan Region (SPMR) remains at unhealthy levels (CETESB, 1998). The most significant air quality problems are related to PM less than 10 microns in diameter (PM_{10}), and photochemical smog or O_3. Nitrogen dioxide (NO_2) and CO concentrations also exceed healthy levels on some days. SO_2 has been reduced to acceptable levels.

PM

Annual average PM_{10} concentrations in the SPMR in 1998 ranged from $85\mu g/m^3$ in Guarulhos to about $40\mu g/m^3$ in Mauá (CETESB, 1998). The Brazilian air quality standard of $50\mu g/m^3$ for annual average PM_{10} concentrations was exceeded at about half of the monitoring sites. The average SPMR-wide PM_{10} concentration was slightly more than $50\mu g/m^3$ in 1998, and has been significantly higher in the recent past – reaching $75\mu g/m^3$ in 1994 and 1995 and about $60\mu g/m^3$ in 1997.

In the SPMR, a receptor study carried out by CETESB indicates that about 40 per cent of ambient PM_{10} concentrations are due to PM emitted by motor vehicles, while secondary particles and resuspended dust account for 25 per cent each and industrial processes for the remaining 10 per cent. Since vehicles are also the main sources of particle-forming NO_x, SO_2 and organic emissions, the total vehicular contribution to ambient PM_{10} concentrations is probably around 55 to 60 per cent. Most of this is attributable to diesel vehicles, as direct PM emissions from gasoline vehicles tend to be very low.

Ozone (O_3)

The Brazilian air quality standard for O_3 is $160\mu g/m^3$, with a higher 'attention' level at $200\mu g/m^3$, both on a one-hour average basis. Monitoring data for the SPMR show that the one-hour O_3 concentration standard of $160\mu g/m^3$ is exceeded on 8–10 per cent of the days of the year, while the 'attention' limit of $200\mu g/m^3$ is exceeded on about 2 per cent of the days.

Carbon monoxide

The Brazilian air quality standard for CO is 9ppm for eight hours, and the attention level is 15ppm. Data for 1998 show that the primary CO standard was exceeded in several stations on 2–3 per cent of the days in the year, but the monitored concentrations never reached the attention level. CO concentrations in the SPMR have been decreasing since 1990, due largely to the widespread use of catalytic converters and alcohol fuels.

Nitrogen dioxide

The Brazilian standards for NO_2 include a one-hour standard of $320\mu g/m^3$ and an annual average standard of $100\mu g/m^3$. In 1998, the short term NO_2 standard was exceeded at four monitoring stations in the SPMR, with the greatest number of exceedances amounting to 0.75 per cent of the days in the year. No monitoring stations exceeded the annual average air quality standard of $100\mu g/m^3$. Measured annual average concentrations in 1998 ranged from 30 to $80\mu g/m^3$, with the majority of stations showing levels higher than the 40 to $50\mu g/m^3$ recommended by the World Health Organization (WHO).

Overall summary

The air quality in the SPMR is very poor. In 1998, the average of 24 urban observation points showed that only 45 per cent of the days were classified as attaining good air quality, and 55 per cent were classified as regular or inadequate quality. The average disguises some extreme situations, such as for instance Cubatao-V Parisi, where only 16 per cent of the days were classified as 'good air quality'. In 1983 the air quality standard for CO in Cerqueira Cesar, an observation point assumed to be representative of the SPMR, was exceeded on 100 days. In 1995 it was exceeded on 23 days, and in 1997 on only three days. This evolution shows an improvement in the overall situation.

Transportation as a source of air pollution in Sao Paulo

The transportation system is responsible for almost the total emissions of CO, HC and NO_x and is a significant source of PM.

The SPMR's total number of vehicles in 1967 was 493,000; in 1997, 3.1 million vehicles were registered. This evolution (a yearly average rate of growth of 9.6 per cent) is much higher than the rate of population growth (1.7 per cent per annum between 1990 and 2000). Sixty-nine per cent of the vehicles use gasoline, 24 per cent use alcohol and 6 per cent use diesel.

Vehicle emission regulations

Brazil was the first country in South America to adopt regulations to control motor vehicle emissions. In 1976 the National Traffic Council (CONTRAN – Conselho Nacional de Trânsito) established control over gaseous and vapour emissions from engine crankcases. In the same year the government of the state of Sao Paulo established the limit of Ringelmann 2 as the emission standard for in-use diesel vehicles. The same set of regulations required that new light duty vehicles (LDVs) would have to attain emission limits for CO, HCs and NO_x before being sold to the public, and used the US FTP 75 test methodology to certify the attainment of the limits. These requirements were set by the Sao Paulo State Environmental Protection Agency (CETESB – Companhia de Tecnologia de Saneamento Ambiental), based on the US approach to controlling vehicular emissions, which was considered to be the most advanced at that time. Unfortunately, due to the lack of background information on pollutant emissions, no emissions limits were established. Although this resulted in ineffective regulation, it opened the doors to emissions evaluation research.

At that time the federal Special Secretary for the Environment (Secretaria Especial do Meio Ambiente, SEMA) had no mandate to control pollutant emissions from motor vehicles, so all issues regarding this subject were the responsibility of CONTRAN.

In 1977 CONTRAN enacted Resolution 510, which required diesel vehicles to attain the Ringelmann 2 standard nationwide. For locations at altitudes higher than 500m the more lenient Ringelmann 3 standard was used.

CETESB and representatives of the Brazilian Motor Vehicle Manufacturers Association started to debate and negotiate over the basis for the implementation of a control programme. The federal government joined these discussions through the newly established National Institute of Standards, Metrology and Industrial Quality (Instituto Nacional de Metrologia, Normalização e Qualidade Industrial, INMETRO) and through Petrobras, the state oil company. The discussions resulted in the first technical reference document – Standard NBR 6601 – which became effective in 1981 and described in detail the test procedure to be used for LDV emissions measurement. Although the standard was based on the US EPA 75 procedure, it had a few changes due to the characteristics of Brazilian fuels (ie gasohol and ethanol). Following this standard, others were drawn up to cover different topics such as test fuel specifications and analytical procedures. With regard to heavy duty vehicles (HDVs), the test procedures adopted by ABNT (Associação Brasileira de Normas Técnicas) were based on the European standards, because most Brazilian HDV manufacturers have a European background and it was thought that it would be more appropriate and cost-effective to follow European experience in emissions control for this class of vehicles.

In 1981 Congress created the National Environment Council (Conselho Nacional do Meio Ambiente, CONAMA) and placed SEMA within the structure of the Office of the President. By law CONAMA was given the exclusive right to establish emissions control requirements for motor vehicles, and SEMA was given the status and power to develop and implement pollution control policies. Within this framework, SEMA became the coordinating and enforcement institution and CONAMA the regulating body. The law also created a new institute responsible for the management of natural resources (Instituto Nacional do Meio Ambiente e dos Recursos Naturais Renováveis, IBAMA), which years later would be restructured and incorporate some of SEMA's responsibilities.

With the establishment of a federal structure to deal with motor vehicle pollution this subject gained more importance and CETESB was officially asked to become technical assistant to SEMA and represent the federal government in negotiations with the automotive industry. This combination proved to be very effective because it made used of technical expertise and governmental representation. Nevertheless, progress was slow because the automotive industry and Petrobras were reluctant to make investments, and used the same arguments presented by their counterparts from the US and Europe in the 1960s and 1970s to postpone emissions control regulations. However, in this case there was a difference: while in the US and Europe the discussions were influenced by uncertainties regarding the availability, efficacy, durability and cost of the emissions control systems that were in the process of being developed and tested, the situation in Brazil was more focused on the economics and applicability of these systems.

In 1985 both ANFAVEA and CETESB prepared emissions regulation proposals. While ANFAVEA's proposal was rejected because it was considered too lenient, CETESB's was approved by the governor of Sao Paulo and was sent to the president, who asked SEMA to create a working group and evaluate it. After intensive negotiations in which the Ministry of Industry and Commerce defended the interests of the automotive industry, the environmental sector

Table 8.14 *Automotive emissions limits for Brazil for light duty vehicles*

Exhaust emissions	1988	1992	1997
CO g/km	24.0	12.0	2.0
HC g/km	2.1	1.2	0.3
NO$_x$ g/km	2.0	1.4	0.6
Aldehydes		0.15	0.03
PM		0.5	0.5
CO idle %	3.0	2.5	0.5
HC idle ppm	600	400	250
Fuel evaporation (g/test)	–	6.0	6.0
Crankcase	Zero	Zero	Zero

Note: diesel passenger cars are prohibited.

agreed to soften the proposal. A new consensus proposal was prepared and the national motor vehicle emissions control programme (Programa de Controle da Poluição por Veículos Automotores, PROCONVE) was created.

Since then, PROCONVE has been gradually implemented and improved. It is based on a complex set of about 40 regulatory requirements that followed the first resolution. The metrological certification activities related to tests and measurements are the responsibility of INMETRO, which follows resolutions set by the National Council of Metrology, Standardization and Industrial Quality (Conselho Nacional de Metrologia, Normalização e Qualidade Industrial, CONMETRO). These resolutions are established in agreement with CETESB, IBAMA and CONAMA.

There are ongoing discussions between the government and the automotive industry about emissions control requirements for the next ten years.

The role of CETESB is to work closely with IBAMA under a formal agreement. CETESB's obligations include the evaluation of emissions certification requests, research activities, proposals for new regulations and revisions of the existing regulations, technical assistance and general support.

Table 8.15 *Heavy duty vehicles (grams per kilowatt hour) (R49 test procedure)*

Effective date*	CO	HC	NO$_x$	PM
1/1/94	4.9	1.2	9.0	0.7/0.4**
1/1/96	4.9	1.2	9.0	0.7/0.4**
1/1/98	4.0	1.1	7.0	0.15

Notes: * = 0.7 for engines below 85kW; 0.4 for engines above.
** = The phase-in schedule for urban buses and domestically produced engines is slower.

CONCLUSIONS

While developing countries currently have very few motorized vehicles per capita compared with the OECD countries, the vehicle population is growing very rapidly. Further, the mix of vehicles, especially the predominance of motorcycles and scooters with highly polluting two-stroke engines, is unique and emits substantially more pollution per kilometre driven than is typical in the OECD countries. Most of the current vehicle population is concentrated in the major cities, with the result that these cities are already highly polluted. As a result of these pollutants there are serious health problems, especially among the very old, the very young and those least able to cope.

Significant progress is being made, however. Taiwan has been implementing an aggressive motorcycle control programme that has 2003 as the expected date for elimination of new two-stroke motorcycles. Further, they are rapidly expanding the conversion to electric motorcycles. A number of other Asian countries, including Thailand and China, are expected to follow Taiwan's lead in cleaning up motorcycles. Singapore has developed one of the pre-eminent land transport planning programmes in the world serving as a model for its neighbours. Sao Paulo is also moving forwards with tight vehicle standards.

Many developing countries have made or will soon make progress to reduce vehicle emissions as a major source of air pollution in cities. For example, Thailand banned all sales of leaded gasoline in 1996 and China and India followed in 2000. All new cars sold in Brazil, Hong Kong, Singapore, Taiwan, Thailand and South Korea have been required to be equipped with catalytic converters for several years, and China, India and the Philippines recently followed suit.

While there is some reason for optimism, there is also great cause for concern as vehicle populations continue to grow rapidly and to be concentrated in megacities, which are increasingly spread across the region. Fundamental shifts to inherently clean transport technologies such as fuel cells and electric vehicles are gaining increased attention.

REFERENCES

Beijing Municipal Environment Protection Bureau (1999) *Urban Transport and Environment in Beijing*, Beijing Municipal Environment Protection Bureau/Beijing Municipal Public Security and Traffic Administration Bureau/Beijing Urban Planning, Design and Research Academy, Beijing

California EPA (1998) *Proposed Identification of Diesel Exhaust as a Toxic Air Contaminant, Appendix III Part A: Exposure Assessment,* California Environmental Protection Agency/California Air Resources Board, Sacramento

CETESB (1998) Relatorio de Qualidade do Ar no Estado de Sao Paulo: 1998, CETESB, Sao Paulo

Health Effects Institute (1995) *Diesel Exhaust: A Critical Analysis of Emissions, Exposure, and Health Effects*, Health Effects Institute, Boston

IARC (1982) 'Some industrial chemicals and dyestuffs' in *Monographs on the Evaluation of Carcinogenic Risk of Chemicals to Humans*, vol 29, International Agency for Research on Cancer, Lyon, pp345–389

IARC (1989) 'Diesel and gasoline engine exhausts and some nitroarenes' in *Monographs on the Evaluation of Carcinogenic Risk of Chemicals to Humans*, vol 46, International Agency for Research on Cancer, Lyon

IARC (1995) 'Formaldehyde' in *Wood Dust and Formaldehyde*, Monographs on the Carcinogenic Risks to Humans, vol 62, International Agency for Research on Cancer, Lyon, pp217–362

Lumley, M, Barker, H and Murray, J A (1990) 'Benzene in petrol' in *Lancet*, vol 336, pp1318–1319

MATES II study, www.aqmd.gov/news1/MATES_II_results.htm

Ministry of Surface Transport, New Delhi, India, personal communication

National Institute for Occupational Safety and Health (1988) 'Carcinogenic effects of exposure to diesel exhaust' in *NIOSH Current Intelligence Bulletin 50 DHHS*, NIOSH Publication No 88–116, Center for Disease Control, Atlanta, GA

Professor He Kebin, Tsinghua University, personal communication

Shanghai Municipal Government (1999) *Strategy for Sustainable Development of Urban Transportation and Environment for a Metropolis with Coordinating Development of Transportation and Environment Toward the 21st Century*, Shanghai Municipal Government, Shanghai

Taiwan EPA, Taipei, Taiwan, personal communication

United Nations (2002) *World Urbanization Prospects: The 2001 Revision*, United Nations, New York

US EPA (1985) *Interim Quantitative Cancer Unit Risk Estimates Due to Inhalation of Benzene*, prepared by the Office of Health and Environmental Assessment, Carcinogen Assessment Group, Washington, DC for the Office of Air Quality Planning and Standards, Washington, DC

US EPA (1985) *Mutagenicity and Carcinogenicity Assessment of 1,3-Butadiene*, EPA/600/8–85/004F, US Environmental Protection Agency, Office of Health and Environmental Assessment, Washington, DC

US EPA (1987) *Health Assessment Document for Acetaldehyde – External Review Draft*, Report No EPA 600/8–86/015A, Office of Health and Environmental Assessment, Research Triangle Park, NC

US EPA (1993) *Environmental Protection Agency, Integrated Risk Information System (IRIS)*, Office of Health and Environmental Assessment, Environmental Criteria and Assessment Office, Cincinnati, OH

US EPA (1993) *Air Quality Criteria for Oxides of Nitrogen*, EPA/600/8–91/049aF, Washington, DC

US EPA (1993) *Motor Vehicle-Related Air Toxics Study*, EPA Report No EPA 420–R–93–005, US Environmental Protection Agency, Office of Mobile Sources, Ann Arbor, MI

US EPA (1995) *Review of National Ambient Air Quality Standards for Nitrogen Dioxide, Assessment of Scientific and Technical Information*, OAQPS Staff Paper, EPA–452/R–95–005

US EPA (1996) *Air Quality Criteria for Ozone and Related Photochemical Oxidants*, EPA/600/P–93/004aF

US EPA (1996) *Review of National Ambient Air Quality Standards for Ozone, Assessment of Scientific and Technical Information*, OAQPS Staff Paper, EPA–452/R–96–007

US EPA (1996) *Air Quality Criteria for Particulate Matter*, EPA/600/P–95/001aF

US EPA (1998) *Environmental Protection Agency, Carcinogenic Effects of Benzene: An Update*, EPA/600/P–97/001F, National Center for Environmental Assessment, Washington, DC

US EPA (1999) *Analysis of the Impacts of Control Programs on Motor Vehicle Toxic Emissions and Exposure in Urban Areas and Nationwide: Volume I*, EPA420–R–99–029

US EPA (1999) *Environmental Protection Agency, Integrated Risk Information System (IRIS)*, Office of Health and Environmental Assessment, Environmental Criteria and Assessment Office, Cincinnati, OH

US EPA (1999) 'Slope factor for 1,3-butadiene', memo from Dr Aparna Koppikar, ORD-NCEA to Laura McKlevey, OAQPS and Pamela Brodowicz, OMS, April 26

US EPA (1999) *Air Quality Criteria For Carbon Monoxide*, Second External Review Draft, US Environmental Protection Agency

US EPA (2002) *Health Assessment Document for Diesel Engine Exhaust*, USEPA EPA/600/8-90/057F, US Environmental Protection Agency, Office of Research and Development, National Center for Environmental Assessment, Washington, DC

Peter Wiederker, OECD, personal communication

World Health Organization (1996) *Diesel Fuel and Exhaust Emissions: International Program on Chemical Safety*, World Health Organization, Geneva

World Health Organization (2000) *Air Quality Guidelines for Europe,* Second Edition, WHO Regional Office for Europe, Copenhagen

Yu Xiaoxuan, Beijing Environmental Protection Bureau, personal communication

9

Air Quality in Hong Kong and the Impact of Pollution on Health 1988–1997

Anthony Johnson Hedley, Chit-Ming Wong, Tai-Hing Lam, Sarah Morag McGhee and Stefan Ma

ABSTRACT

Hong Kong's air quality is similar in many ways to that of other capitals and major urban centres around the world; therefore, epidemiological studies in Hong Kong may contribute to the global evidence on the relationship between air pollution and health. This chapter summarizes some studies of air pollution and impacts on health in Hong Kong, as they may provide an indication of impacts in other similar cities. The studies found that overall, the relative risks for health effects of pollution, including admissions for all respiratory disease, asthma and lung disease, showed higher excess risks for all age groups than results for Western European cities using similar methodologies. Similar findings were made for hospital deaths.

Pollution is now responsible for eroding the previously gained economic advantages of Asia, which have resulted in improved population health. However, policy-makers can be confident that controls on pollution sources will, in addition to arresting degradation of the environment, bring about measurable improvements in health, particularly in children and the elderly. Pollution controls will reduce premature deaths in the chronically sick and elderly and thereby reduce avoidable morbidity and mortality and associated hospital costs.

BACKGROUND

There has been increasing awareness in the Hong Kong Special Administrative Region (HKSAR) over the past ten years that air pollution is degrading the quality of the environment and affecting the health of citizens of all ages.

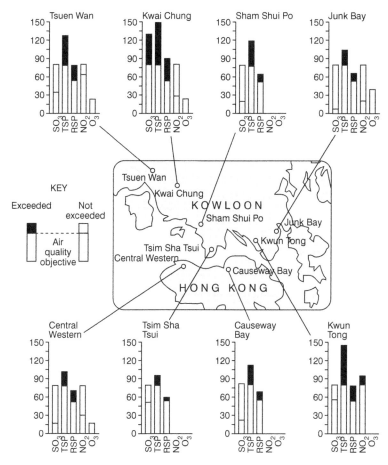

Notes:
1   Figures shown are annual average concentrations
2   All concentrations are in μg/m³
3   Annual average pollutant concentrations are in grey
4   Exceedence of annual average air quality objective (ACO) are in black

Figure 9.1 *Hong Kong's average pollutant concentrations recorded at air quality monitoring stations during 1988*

In 1988, exceedances of air quality objectives (AQOs) were common (Environmental Protection Department, 1989) and the Environmental Protection Department received over 2000 complaints about air quality in the late 1980s and early 1990s (Figure 9.1).

In July 1990 the Air Pollution Control (Fuel Restriction) Regulation became law. This prohibited the use of fuel oil containing more than 0.5 per cent by weight of sulphur (Hong Kong Government, 1990). There was an immediate decrease in ambient concentrations of sulphur dioxide (SO_2) by over 80 per cent in the most polluted districts (Figure 9.2) (Environmental Protection Department, 1991, 1992, 1993). Sulphate concentrations in respirable suspended particulates (RSP) also fell by up to 35 per cent.

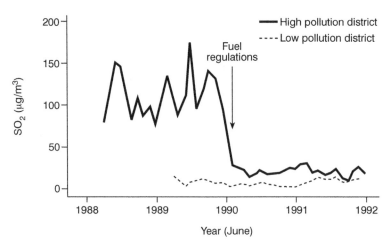

Figure 9.2 *Changes in SO₂ following the 1990 fuel regulations*

Levels of other pollutants such as nitrogen oxides (NO_x), particulates and ozone (O_3) were unchanged following this intervention. Lower levels of SO_2 were maintained but overall air quality has deteriorated and, in 1997, exceedances of nitrogen dioxide (NO_2) and RSP occurred at six out of nine air quality monitoring stations located in different districts of the HKSAR (Table 9.1) (Government of the Hong Kong Special Administrative Region, 1998).

Hong Kong's air quality is similar in many ways to that of other capitals and major urban centres around the world; therefore, the epidemiological studies in the HKSAR may contribute to the global evidence on the relationship between air pollution and health. It is clear that the status of a city may be categorized in different ways by different pollutants, assuming that the measurements are comparable. In comparison with other Asian cities, Hong Kong ranks middling to low for ambient concentrations of SO_2 and carbon monoxide (CO) and, for particulates, it has lower ambient concentrations than Taipei, Shanghai and Guangzhou but higher than Seoul, Tokyo and Singapore. Hong Kong has higher ambient O_3 concentrations than Kuala Lumpur, Tokyo and Singapore but lower concentrations than the Chinese cities of Guangzhou and Taipei (Government of the Hong Kong Special Administrative Region, 1998). In 1999 Hong Kong's pollution made international headlines as tourists observed visibility dropping to 3000m and once famous views disappearing. In a series of different studies, variations in air pollutants by both geographical zone and time have been used to measure the impact of pollution on health and, where possible, the effects of intervention. This chapter reviews some of the more pertinent studies, but a consideration of methods is needed to properly appreciate the results.

Table 9.1 *Compliance with air quality objectives in 1997 in nine districts of Hong Kong, for O_3, NO_2 and RSP*

Station	1 hour	1 hour	24 hour	1 year	24 hour	1 year
1	✔	✔	✗	✔	✔	✗
2	✔	✔	✔	✔	✔	✔
3	✔	✔	✔	✔	✔	✔
4	✔	✔	✔	✔	✔	✗
5	–	✔	✗	✔	✔	✗
6	✔	✔	✔	✔	✔	✗
7	✔	✔	✔	✔	✔	✗
8	✔	✔	✔	✔	✔	✔
9	–	✗	✗	✗	✔	✗

Source: modified from Government of the Hong Kong Special Administrative Region, 1998
Notes: ✔ = Complied
✗ = Not complied
– = Not available

METHODS

Measurements of health in children

Respiratory symptoms

Children are the most sensitive members of the general population to the health effects of air pollution. Studies of the impact of pollution on health have been based on comparisons of the health of primary school children, aged mainly eight to ten years, in two districts with higher and lower levels of pollution. Children were sampled from schools considered to be located in constituencies that were representative of the air quality in the two districts (Ong et al, 1991). Data were collected by standardized questionnaires from children and parents who were asked about respiratory symptoms including coughs, phlegm, wheezing, sore throats, nasal problems and doctor-diagnosed asthma. Questions were also asked about smoking and how many categories of people (father, mother, siblings, other relatives or lodgers) smoked in the family home, parental educational attainment, occupational status and the use of domestic fuels, incense and mosquito coils. The response rate ranged from 96 per cent (parents) up to 99 per cent (children). In the first year of the survey, before the introduction of new fuel regulations in the territory, 3521 children took part, 1504 in the low pollution district and 2017 in the high pollution district.

Bronchial reactivity

An abnormal tendency for the pulmonary airways to narrow when challenged with an aerosol of the compound histamine is a characteristic of individuals with asthma. This reaction is followed by a fall in lung function which can be measured with a meter. This response, called bronchial hyper-responsiveness, can be observed in well children and may reflect sensitization by exposure to environmental factors such as chemical pollutants, biological allergens, pollen or house dust mites. This test was used to examine whether there was any variation in bronchial reactivity between children with higher or lower levels of exposure to air pollution.

The children were examined and tested on two occasions, in 1989 and 1990, before the introduction of the fuel regulations and again on two occasions, in 1991 and 1992, after the intervention.

Measures of health in adults

A well population of workers

A comprehensive health enquiry was conducted in a young adult public sector workforce (mean age around 32 years) with responsibilities either outdoors at street level, indoors in offices or in marine environments. Information obtained included current respiratory symptoms and a detailed history of both active and passive smoking (Department of Community Medicine, 1997).

Measurement of lung function

Representative samples of individuals in the workforce who were engaged in street level outdoor activities took part in lung function testing sessions before and after eight-hour shifts. In this survey the test was used to determine whether lung function was impaired by a normal working shift, usually of eight hours, at street level.

Variation in population health by ambient air pollution

In order to take a whole population approach to the estimation of possible variations in health caused by air pollution, statistical modelling techniques were used to analyse patterns of daily hospital admissions to public sector hospitals and hospital deaths in relation to daily variations in pollutants.

The sources of information included the integrated patient administration system and medical records abstracting system associated with the public sector hospital service and the Environmental Protection Department database of daily ambient pollutant concentrations. The pollutants included in the analyses were NO_2, RSP measured as PM_{10}, O_3 and SO_2.

The statistical modelling techniques were based on the protocols used by the European collaborating group known as APHEA (Air Pollution on Health: a European Approach) (Katsouyanni et al, 1996).

FINDINGS

Respiratory health of children

Inferences about the effects of air pollution on children's health were drawn from two sources: a cross-sectional survey, and a cohort follow-up study which spanned the introduction of the new fuel regulations.

Table 9.2 *Crude prevalence ratios (%) for respiratory symptoms before and after the introduction of restrictions on fuel sulphur content in districts with lower and higher pollution*

Respiratory symptoms		1989	1990	1991
Coughs/sore throats	S:	16.1	13.9	11.7
	K:	19.8	16.8	11.1
Phlegm	S:	16.8	13.2	9.4
	K:	19.2	14.2	8.1
Wheezing	S:	11.3	10.5	9.2
	K:	12.7	11.2	9.3
Nasal symptoms	S:	35.6	31	32.6
	K:	38.1	31.4	32.4

Notes: S = Southern district (lower pollution).
K = Kwai Tsing (higher pollution).

Respiratory symptoms

In 1989 and 1990, after adjustment for potential confounding factors (such as smoking in the home), significant excess risks for reported coughs, sore throats, wheezing with asthmatic symptoms and wheezing alone were found in the most polluted district (Peters et al, 1996). The frequencies of all the respiratory symptoms were highest among the youngest children (aged eight years), higher in boys than girls and higher in children living in the most polluted district. Children who lived in homes where smoking took place also had a higher prevalence of symptoms.

Over a three-year period the prevalence ratios declined in both districts (Table 9.2). Apart from the prevalence of nasal symptoms including allergic rhinitis and sinusitis, there was an apparently greater drop in the district with the higher level of pollution. After adjustment for potential confounding factors, the finding of significant excess risks in the most polluted district had disappeared by 1991 (Figure 9.3a, b), although there were some apparent residual effects (Department of Community Medicine, 1993).

In contrast, the observed effects of exposure to environmental tobacco smoke at home, with excess risks for coughs or sore throats and phlegm, were unchanged after the intervention of the fuel regulations (Figure 9.3c).

Bronchial responsiveness

The differences in the prevalence of bronchial hyper-responsiveness between districts were studied to assess the effectiveness of the intervention. In the pre-intervention period, children in the higher pollution district had a higher prevalence of hyper-responsiveness (Tam et al, 1994). In the cohort of children who were followed up after the introduction of the fuel regulations, a decline in bronchial hyper-responsiveness over a two-year period was observed, with the rate of decline in hyper-responsiveness greater in the most polluted district (Wong et al, 1998) (Table 9.3).

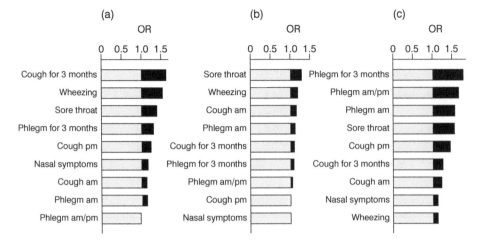

OR = odds ratio

Figure 9.3 *Odds ratios and excess risks (black) for nine respiratory symptoms in primary school children associated with exposure to ambient air pollution before (a) and after (b) the introduction of restrictions on the sulphur content of fuel. The excess risks associated with living in a smoking home (c) were unchanged by the intervention*

Costs and benefits of air quality improvement

The information gained from the children's respiratory health survey was used to carry out an economic appraisal of the costs and benefits of the government's intervention based on the fuel regulations. The analysis, which was principally based on the valuation of avoided doctor consultations, concluded that Hong Kong (its citizens and policy-makers) implicitly valued the non-monetized benefits higher than the net costs. In addition, a portion of the intervention costs were offset by the avoidance of acute respiratory symptoms and healthcare utilization (Barron et al, 1995).

Health effects in adults

A healthy workforce

The types of duties in the workforce studied were used as proxy indicators for exposure to ambient pollution. The frequencies of coughs, phlegm and wheezing were used as the health outcome measure. Workers who were engaged in duties at street level experienced significantly increased excess risks for coughing and the production of phlegm compared with workers in a marine environment. Similarly, when outdoor workers were compared with those with indoor administrative duties, they had significant excess risks for coughing, phlegm and wheezing (Table 9.4).

Table 9.3 *Prevalence of bronchial hyper-responsiveness before (1990) and after (1991–1992) the introduction of restrictions on fuel sulphur content in districts with lower and higher pollution levels*

Year	Prevalence (%) of bronchial hyper-responsiveness before and after air quality intervention		
District	1990	1991	1992
Lower pollution	30.6	17.8	10.9
Higher pollution	22.7	11.1	12.0

The results, which were adjusted for all factors that might influence health (such as gender, marital status, education level, smoking and exposure to passive smoking), suggest that outdoor shift work is associated with several bronchitic symptoms in this urban environment.

These findings are supported by the results of lung function tests, which showed that in the non-smoking subjects who spent the longest periods on the streets, at the kerbside, during shift work, the pre- and post-shift lung function tests indicated a significant drop after an eight-hour shift (Department of Community Medicine, 1997).

Pollution effects on hospital admissions

Reports from other centres based on analyses of daily hospital admission data have shown significant variations in admissions for cardiovascular and respiratory disease by variations in ambient daily pollutant concentrations. In Hong Kong, a sub-tropical environment, time trends, seasonality and weather conditions explained 31–79 per cent of the variations in all the health outcomes under study. In Hong Kong, as in temperate zones, cardiovascular mortality is strongly associated with lower temperatures in the cool season (Wong et al, 1999b). In addition, all of the four pollutants that were studied showed a significant association with daily hospital admissions for cardiovascular and respiratory diseases, both combined and separately. The excess risks were in the range of 3–10 per cent (Wong et al, 1998). The effects of pollutants on circulatory and respiratory diseases were stronger for older age groups, with significant excess risks of 5–10 per cent in those aged 65 or over. Both NO_2 and O_3 were strongly associated with hospital deaths from cardiovascular and respiratory diseases.

Table 9.4 *Excess risks for coughs and production of phlegm for workers who were engaged in duties at street level*

	Cough	Phlegm
Work environment	Excess risk	Excess risk
Street level versus marine workers	49% p<0.0001	17% p=0.0235
Outdoors versus indoors	57% p=0.0002	32% p=0.0082

Note: p = probability

Concentrations of O_3 in Hong Kong increased more than 80 per cent between 1993 and 2000, the hourly air quality objective of $24\mu g/m^3$ being frequently violated. In an analysis of approximately 87,000 daily hospital admissions for circulatory diseases through accident and emergency departments in the over-65 age group between January 1995 and June 1997, there was a significant excess risk of admission for all circulatory diseases, dysrhythmias and heart failure. A significant interaction with season was observed, with excess risks much increased in the cool season (Wong et al, 1999a). Overall, the relative risks for the health effects of pollution, including admissions for all respiratory diseases, asthma and chronic obstructive pulmonary disease, showed higher excess risks for all age groups when compared with the pooled results of Western European cities from the APHEA studies. Similar findings were made for hospital deaths.

Using similar databases and identical methodology, we recently completed a comparison between the cities of Hong Kong and London in terms of daily hospital admissions and their associations with air pollutant concentrations. We demonstrated significant positive associations for respiratory admissions in those aged 65 years and over with PM_{10}, NO_2, SO_2 and O_3 in both cities. Associations were stronger in the cool season in Hong Kong and in the warmer season in London, during which levels of humidity are at their lowest in each city.

For all cardiac admissions at all ages, in both cities, significant positive associations (stronger in the cool season) were observed for PM_{10}, NO_2 and SO_2. Patterns of association with ischaemic heart disease in the two cities were similar. The results clearly indicate that despite the differences in climate, social lifestyle and other environmental factors, air pollution is a cause of detrimental health effects and increased healthcare utilization and costs (Wong et al, 2002).

These findings are supported by a separate study of all causes of mortality based on registered deaths occurring both within and outside the hospital system. We found significant effects during the cool season for the oxidant pollutants NO_2, SO_2 and O_3 on cardiovascular, respiratory and all-causes mortality. The effects of the oxidant pollutants were stronger than those associated with PM_{10}, although this was significant for respiratory mortality. We concluded that although there is clear evidence for the harm caused by RSP, in this sub-tropical city environmental controls must take account of the fact that oxidant pollutants and their sources may be more important than particulates (Wong et al, 2001).

DISCUSSION

The evidence available from both well-population epidemiological surveys and analyses of databases for air pollutants and records of hospitalized patients indicates consistent and strong associations between variations in ambient air pollutants and bad health outcomes. The evidence suggests that both past and current air quality objectives have not protected several large sections of the Hong Kong community from air pollution-related health problems, including particularly the very young, the sick and the elderly.

The findings from a wide spectrum of different types of enquiries show that, whereas specific benefits can be gained from the reduction of one particular pollutant, in this case SO_2, all the pollutants measured are associated with adverse health effects. It follows from this that policy-makers must focus on the *sources* of pollution rather than individual pollutant species.

In Hong Kong, government proposals to reduce ambient air pollution include the conversion of all light commercial diesel road vehicles to run on liquefied petroleum gas (LPG). Exhaust emissions from LPG vehicles would be lower for CO and hydrocarbons and markedly lower for NO_x and particulates compared with diesel. The choice of LPG has been made because legislators rejected an earlier proposal for a diesel to petrol (gasoline) switch. However, the timescale for the conversion extends up to the year 2005 and this is now the subject of a vigorous public debate in Hong Kong. The short term conversion of all taxis to LPG power units would cost about US$770m, but would eliminate a large source of pollutants very rapidly.

Other government interventions include the routine roadside measurement of smoke emissions, the calling in of 30,000 vehicles per year which are reported by 'spotters' and the phasing out of leaded petrol in 2000. This is a generally inefficient approach because fines do not remove heavily polluting vehicles from the road. Given the evidence of detriment to the health of the population, the licences of these vehicles should be removed.

The adverse health effects of pollution have been measurable over the past ten years. Epidemiological evidence of harm to health, derived from local studies, has been used to evaluate and support action by the Environmental Protection Department and strengthen arguments for legislative action. However, public expressions of concern and a growing intolerance of the present situation have been closely related to the visible and other sensory effects of ambient pollution. Hong Kong has lost its horizon, and the aesthetic impact on the environment and quality of life has been an important factor in making the community call for action. There are indications that the situation is improving, but population growth and slow progress towards clean transportation will present major challenges to air quality control.

All of the analyses that relate morbidity and mortality patterns to ambient levels of NO_2, SO_2, RSP and O_3 show excess risks for health problems, hospital admissions and hospital mortality. On the basis of these findings, it can be predicted that progressive reductions in current levels of pollution would benefit large numbers in the population. Caution must be exercised in the interpretation of the outputs of models. Environmentalists, the media and possibly policy-makers want estimates of 'body counts'. However, it is not possible to estimate precisely the excess numbers of admissions or deaths with the methods used. It can only be concluded that variations in pollution probably cause or aggravate health problems. This is at least consistent with the findings in well-population subjects that marked variations in the frequency of symptoms are associated with pollution, which is a good indicator that people are being adversely exposed. In the case of hospital admissions and deaths, it was found that pollutant concentrations are related to acute events (admissions and deaths) for conditions such as coronary heart disease and chronic lung disease, which show an excess over predicted levels whereas outcomes related to cancer do not. We have recently confirmed this in new analyses of mortality data in the years following the introduction of low sulphur fuel. The principal benefit was a reduction in deaths due to respiratory and cardiac disease (Hedley et al, 2001).

Any strategy to reduce the risk of cardiovascular and respiratory disease and premature death requires an inter-sectoral approach. The risks from tobacco for those exposed, including passive smoking in children, are much greater than those from air pollution. Air pollution, on the other hand, now affects everyone in the community and its effects tend to negate the benefits of rapid social and economic development, which ironically have created the pollution.

Hong Kong could have acted on more stringent pollution controls at least a decade ago, but a non-interventionist government philosophy prevailed. A lack of good quality data on the health effects of pollution contributed to this. We must strengthen epidemiological and economic research and clinical analyses of the impact of air pollution on health to aid rapid progress towards better environmental controls.

The present situation clearly signals that the dominance of diesel vehicles in the commercial sector and other aspects of current transportation policies are unsustainable. Nevertheless, the trend in infrastructural developments is to build highways rather than other mass transit systems. The Hong Kong experience indicates that this will be associated with further degradation of air quality and adverse effects on health, tourism and general perceptions of quality of life.

CONCLUSIONS

- Pollution is now responsible for eroding the economic advantages of Asia, for example in terms of improved population health and tourism.
- Policy-makers can be confident that controls on pollution sources will, in addition to arresting the degradation of the environment, bring about measurable improvements in health, particularly in children and the elderly.
- Pollution controls will reduce premature deaths in the chronically sick and elderly and thereby reduce avoidable morbidity and mortality and associated hospital costs.
- The response time for measurable health benefits to be realized is short, measured in weeks and months rather than years. However, the lead time for policy decisions to take effect is likely to be much longer.
- The solution to air pollution in Hong Kong and China must include a new and radical approach to transportation policy, but vested interests and bureaucratic positions on this issue are difficult to change. The prospects for a reduction in the rate of increase in personal forms of transport and a major shift to cleaner forms of mass transport are not promising.

REFERENCES

Barron, W F, Liu, J, Lam, T H, Wong, C M, Peters, J and Hedley, A J (1995) 'Costs and benefits of air quality improvement in Hong Kong' in *Contemporary Economic Policy*, vol 9, pp105–116

Department of Community Medicine (1997) *Health of the Hong Kong Police*, Department of Community Medicine, University of Hong Kong, Hong Kong

Department of Community Medicine (1993) *Air Pollution and Respiratory Health in Hong Kong, 1989–1992*, Report to the Environmental Protection Department, Hong Kong Government, Hong Kong

Environmental Protection Department, *Air Quality in Hong Kong 1986–1996*, CD-ROM, Government Printer, Hong Kong

Environmental Protection Department (1989) *Environment Hong Kong 1989*, Government Printer, Hong Kong

Environmental Protection Department (1991) *Environment Hong Kong 1991: A Review of 1990*, Government Printer, Hong Kong

Environmental Protection Department (1992) *Environment Hong Kong 1992: A Review of 1991*, Government Printer, Hong Kong

Environmental Protection Department (1993) *Environment Hong Kong 1993: A Review of 1992*, Government Printer, Hong Kong

Government of the Hong Kong Special Administrative Region (1998) *A Proposal to Introduce LPG Taxis*, consultation paper, Government of Hong Kong, Hong Kong

Hedley, A J, Wong, C M, Thach, T Q, Chau, P, Lam, T H and Anderson, H R (2001) 'Reduction in both seasonal mortality and longer term mortality trends following restrictions on the sulphur content of fuel oil in Hong Kong', Joint Conference of the International Epidemiological Association and the Society for Social Medicine, 12–15 September, Oxford

Hong Kong Government (1990) 'Air Pollution Control (Fuel Restriction) Regulations 1990' in *Air Pollution Control Ordinance (Chapter 311) Gazette*, vol 4/1990, Government Printer, Hong Kong

Hospital Authority of Hong Kong (2000) *Overview of the HA IT/IS Strategy (1992–2000)*, www.ha.org.hk/it/pcp5.htm

Katsouyanni, K, Schwartz, J, Spix, C, Touloumi, G, Zmirou, D, Zanobetti, A, Wojtyniak, B, Vonk, J M, Tobias, A, Ponka, A, Medina, S, Bacharova, L and Anderson, H R (1996) 'Short term effects of air pollution on health: a European approach using epidemiologic time series data. The APHEA protocol' in *Journal of Epidemiology and Community Health*, vol 50, ppS12–18

Ong, S G, Liu, J, Wong, C M, Lam, T H, Tam, A Y C, Daniel, L and Hedley, A J (1991) 'Studies on the respiratory health of primary school children in urban communities of Hong Kong' in *Science of the Total Environment*, vol 106, pp121–135

Peters, J, Hedley, A J, Wong, C M, Lam, T H, Ong, S G, Liu, J and Spiegelhalter, D J (1996) 'Effects of ambient air pollution intervention and environmental tobacco smoke on children's respiratory health in Hong Kong' in *International Journal of Epidemiology*, vol 25, pp821–828

Tam, A Y C, Wong, C M, Lam, T H, Ong, S G, Peters, J and Hedley, A J (1994) 'Bronchial responsiveness in children exposed to atmospheric pollution in Hong Kong' in *Chest*, vol 104, pp1056–1060

Wong, C M, Lam, T H, Peters, J, Hedley, A J, Ong, S G, Tam, A Y C, Liu, J and Spiegelhalter, D J (1998) 'Comparison between two districts of the effects of an air pollution intervention on bronchial responsiveness in primary school children in Hong Kong' in *Journal of Epidemiology and Community Health*, vol 52, pp571–578

Wong, C M, Atkinson, R W, Anderson, H R, Hedley, A J, Ma, S, Chau, P Y K and Lam, T H (2002) 'A tale of two cities: effect of air pollution on hospital admissions in Hong Kong and London compared' in *Environmental Health Perspectives*, vol 110, pp67–77

Wong, C M, Ma, S, Hedley, A J and Lam, T H (1999a) 'Does ozone have any effect on daily hospital admissions for circulatory diseases?' in *Journal of Epidemiology and Community Health*, vol 53, pp580–581

Wong, C M, Ma, S, Lam, T H and Hedley, A J (1999b) 'Coronary artery disease varies seasonably in subtropics' in *British Medical Journal,* vol 319, pp1004

Wong, C M, Ma, S, Hedley, A J and Lam, T H (2001) 'Effect of air pollution on daily mortality in Hong Kong' in *Environmental Health Perspectives*, vol 109, pp335–340

10

Air Pollution and its Impacts on Health in Santiago, Chile

Bart D Ostro[1]

ABSTRACT

With its unique topography and rapid economic expansion, Santiago, Chile currently experiences extremely high concentrations of particulate matter (PM) air pollution. Several epidemiological studies conducted in Santiago suggest associations between PM_{10} and $PM_{2.5}$ (particulate matter less than 10 and 2.5 microns in diameter, respectively) and several adverse health outcomes including premature mortality and urgent care visits for respiratory ailments. The findings of these studies are generally similar in magnitude to those reported in other cities in Latin America and throughout the world. As a consequence, it is reasonable to utilize the local epidemiologic studies and extrapolate the findings from studies in the US, Canada and Europe in an attempt to quantify the health effects of air pollution in Santiago. Health effects were quantified assuming a threshold (ie, no effects) concentration of either $30\mu g/m^3$ PM_{10} (or approximately $15\mu g/m^3$ $PM_{2.5}$, the proposed US Environmental Protection Agency (EPA) standard) or $20\mu g/m^3$ PM_{10}, the European Union-proposed Stage 2 limit value. The results indicate that substantial health effects are associated with current exposures to particulate matter. For example, with $30\mu g/m^3$ as a threshold concentration, current concentrations of particulate matter are associated with about 700 cases of premature mortality (95 per cent confidence interval (CI) = 400–1300), 5000 extra cases of hospitalization for cardiovascular disease and 700,000 more days with acute respiratory symptoms per year. Assuming a threshold of $20\mu g/m^3$ increases the number of cases of premature mortality to 860 (95 per cent CI = 500–1600) and likewise increases the previous morbidity estimates by about 20 per cent. In recognition of the health consequences of air pollution in Santiago, the government has proposed several strategies aimed at reducing PM_{10} from mobile, industrial and residential sources.

INTRODUCTION

Chile has experienced extremely rapid economic growth over the past two decades, with an accompanying increase in automobile ownership and usage. The capital city of Santiago is now home to about 5 million people, roughly a quarter of all Chileans, and about 800,000 motor vehicles. The high air pollution concentrations of PM_{10} and $PM_{2.5}$ in Santiago are primarily a result of emissions from motor vehicles including private cars, taxis and diesel-powered buses. About 50 per cent of the particles come from mobile sources (Comisión Nacional de Medio Ambiente, 2001). Fossil fuel use for energy production, industrial processes and blowing and resuspended dust also contribute to the problem. The city is situated in a basin surrounded by mountains, with fairly stable atmospheric conditions, including low velocity, turbulence and frequency of winds. In the late autumn and winter an inversion layer prevails about 600–900m above the city, preventing the natural dispersion of pollutants and trapping most particles in the valley. Thus, particulate concentrations in Santiago are among the highest observed in any urban area in the world, with an annual average in 1999 of $74\mu g/m^3$ (Comisión Nacional del Medio Ambiente, 2001).

PM air pollution, sometimes referred to as 'dust and soot', is a pollutant to which all of the general population is regularly exposed. PM_{10} is a heterogeneous mixture of chemicals and particle sizes. It includes particles directly emitted into the air such as diesel soot, road or agricultural dust, or as the result of wood burning or manufacturing processes. It is also produced through photochemical reactions among pollution gases such as sulphur or nitrogen oxides produced from fuel combustion. For example, the nitrogen dioxide produced from automobile emissions will be transformed into nitrates, a constituent of $PM_{2.5}$.

This chapter aims to put the air pollution problem in perspective by first describing some of the epidemiological studies conducted in Santiago. Second, the comparability of the results with studies conducted in other parts of Latin America and in the world will be briefly reviewed. Finally, these studies will be utilized to demonstrate the methodology and provide approximate quantitative estimates of the current effects of air pollution in Santiago.

EPIDEMIOLOGIC OVERVIEW

Most of the health evidence on PM_{10} has been derived from observational epidemiological studies of human populations in a variety of geographic (principally urban) locations. Epidemiologic studies provide 'real world' evidence of associations between concentrations of PM and several adverse health outcomes, including mortality, hospital admissions for respiratory disease, emergency room visits, restricted activity days (including work loss) for adults, upper and lower respiratory symptoms, asthma attacks and the development of acute and chronic bronchitis. These studies typically examine the daily relationship between fluctuations in PM and the various health endpoints (occurring on the same day or several days later), after other potential confounding factors such as temperature, season and day of the week are taken into account. A few of these studies have been conducted in Santiago. The majority, however, have been conducted in different cities and incorporate a wide range of climates, seasonal patterns, chemical compositions of PM and underlying socio-demographics. Thus, extrapolating these findings to Santiago appears reasonable.

Studies of the short term effects of PM exposure typically involve daily time-series observations collected over several months or years. Well designed time-series studies can have several methodological strengths, including:

1   a large sample size (sometimes up to 4–8 years of daily data for an entire city, while at other times approximately 100 people are observed daily over a three month period), conferring substantial statistical power to detect effects;
2   implicit incorporation of a wide range of population demographics, baseline health characteristics and human behaviours, enhancing the generalizability of the results;
3   real world exposures, avoiding the need to extrapolate to lower concentrations or across species;
4   the ability to examine effects in potentially sensitive individuals, children and infants; and
5   a limited number of co-variates or potential confounders, notably other pollutants and weather factors.

Limitations and potential uncertainties associated with time-series studies include:

1   the difficulty in determining actual pollutant concentrations to which people are exposed;
2   the potential for a misclassification of exposure;
3   the potential for the omission of important explanatory factors or the inappropriate control of potential confounding factors;
4   the difficulty in measuring or observing all potential health effects; and
5   co-variation among pollutants making it difficult to attribute an effect to a single pollutant.

Nevertheless, the epidemiological studies of PM provide a major body of evidence regarding the associated health effects and serve as a reasonable basis for attempting to quantify health effects.

STUDIES IN SANTIAGO AND THEIR COMPARABILITY WITH OTHER STUDIES

In recent years several studies have been conducted in Santiago, where there is a robust PM monitoring network operated by the Servicio de Salud Metropolitano del Ambiente. For the most part, this system has been producing daily or near daily measurements of PM_{10} and $PM_{2.5}$ since the early 1990s. In addition, data on sulphur dioxide, nitrogen dioxide, carbon monoxide and ozone are available. Most of the monitors are located near or in the downtown area of the city. The studies include examinations of the effects of short term exposure on mortality and on urgent care visits for respiratory illness.

Mortality associated with acute exposure

Among the first of the studies to use the daily data was an analysis of the association between PM_{10} and daily mortality in Santiago (Ostro et al, 1996). This study used daily data between 1989 and 1991 along with daily counts of mortality from all causes, cardiovascular disease and respiratory disease. In addition, the total daily mortality for men, women and those above age 65 were calculated. After controlling for temperature, hot and cold temperature extremes and season, an association was reported between PM_{10} and all of the different measures of mortality. In the analysis using a Poisson regression model, the results indicated that a $10\mu g/m^3$ change in PM_{10} was associated with a 0.75 per cent (95 per cent CI = 0.5–0.9 per cent) change in daily all-cause mortality. Respiratory-specific mortality was associated with a 1.27 per cent (95 per cent CI = 0.6–1.9 per cent) change per $10\mu g/m^3$ PM_{10}, while for the elderly the association was 0.9 per cent (95 per cent CI = 0.6–1.2 per cent) per $10\mu g/m^3$. Additional sensitivity analysis demonstrated that the association was not unduly influenced by the winter months, the coldest or hottest days, or seasonality in the data.

These findings in Santiago were very consistent with much of the published results for the US, Canada and Europe. Meta-analyses of earlier mortality studies suggest that, after converting the alternative measures of PM used in the original studies to an equivalent PM_{10} concentration, the effects on mortality are fairly consistent (Ostro, 1993; Dockery and Pope, 1994a; Schwartz, 1994a). Specifically, the mean estimated change in daily mortality associated with a one-day $10\mu g/m^3$ change in PM_{10} implied by these studies is approximately 0.8 per cent, with a range of 0.5 per cent to 1.6 per cent. Since these meta-analyses were published, many more studies of short term exposure mortality have been completed. All include control for weather and other potential confounding factors and most use sophisticated smoothing techniques as well. For example, Schwartz et al (1996) examined data from the Harvard six-city studies. This database included monitors that were specifically sited to support ongoing epidemiological studies and be representative of local population exposures. A consistent association was reported between daily mortality and daily exposures to both PM_{10} and $PM_{2.5}$. For PM_{10}, the joint effect estimate was a 0.8 per cent (95 per cent CI = 0.5–1.1) increase in mortality per $10\mu g/m^3$. In another multi-city analysis, Samet et al (2000b) focused on 20 of the largest cities in the US. The combined effect of all of the cities indicated an association within but near the lower end (approximately 0.55 per cent per $10\mu g/m^3$ of PM_{10}) of the range reported by earlier researchers. In addition, the findings for Santiago are consistent with studies from other Latin American cities including Mexico City

(Castillejos et al, 2000) and Sao Paulo, Brazil (Saldiva and Bohm, 1995). Both of these studies reported associations between daily mortality and $PM_{2.5}$. Converting to PM_{10} by multiplying the $PM_{2.5}$ coefficient by 0.55 generates estimates for the two cities of 0.75 per cent and 0.85 per cent per $10\mu g/m^3$, respectively.

In another study of mortality and air pollution in Santiago, Cifuentes et al (2000) examined the impact of $PM_{2.5}$ and coarse particles (CP) (PM_{10}–$PM_{2.5}$) on daily mortality in Santiago from 1988 to 1996. A generalized additive model (GAM) was used to minimize the potentially confounding factors of seasonality and time. Specifically, a locally weighted smooth of time and weather was used to provide a data-driven control for these factors in the regression model. The results indicated that for the full dataset, both $PM_{2.5}$ and CP were associated with all-cause mortality. For example, using a four-day moving average, a $10\mu g/m^3$ change in $PM_{2.5}$ and CP was associated with a 0.8 per cent (95 per cent CI = 0.6–1.1 per cent) and 1.25 per cent (95 per cent CI = 0.8–1.7 per cent) change in mortality, respectively.

For comparison, there are only a few mortality studies currently available using $PM_{2.5}$ and CP, with varying results. For example, Burnett et al (2000) examined mortality and air pollution in eight Canadian cities. The effect of $PM_{2.5}$ on mortality (about 1.2 per cent per $10\mu g/m^3$) was stronger than that of CP (0.71 per cent per $10\mu g/m^3$) with the latter demonstrating a weaker association. In a study of four years of data from Mexico City, CP had a larger impact (4.1 per cent per $\mu g/m^3$) and stronger association than $PM_{2.5}$ (1.5 per cent per $10\mu g/m^3$) for all-cause mortality (Castillejos et al, 2000). Similar results were reported for cardiovascular and respiratory mortality. In a study of Phoenix, Mar et al (2000) found stronger associations of all-cause mortality with CP than with $PM_{2.5}$ for individuals 65 and above, although the magnitude of the effect was greater for $PM_{2.5}$ (2.2 per cent versus 1.2 per cent per $10\mu g/m^3$). Finally, in Detroit, Lippmann et al (2000) examined the effects of different size fractions of PM on mortality. No associations were reported between all-cause mortality and any PM metrics. However, the effect sizes were 1.2 per cent and 1.6 per cent per $10\mu g/m^3$ of $PM_{2.5}$ and CP, respectively. For cardiovascular mortality, associations were reported for CP, but not $PM_{2.5}$. Thus, for mortality associated with specific particle sizes, the findings in Santiago appear to be slightly lower than, but generally consistent with, findings from other studies.

Lower respiratory symptoms

Ostro et al (1999) analysed the association between daily visits to primary healthcare clinics in Santiago, Chile among children under age 2 and ages 2 to 14. Data on respiratory visits to eight clinics in 1992 and 1993 were obtained from the Infant Respiratory Disease Program developed by the Chilean Ministry of Health. These clinics serve about 10 per cent of the child population in the area around Santiago. Using a standardized form, the total number of child medical visits and respiratory morbidity diagnoses were collected every day. Doctors working at each clinic prepared the diagnoses. The researchers of the infant respiratory disease programme trained the record-keeping staff at each clinic to group the diagnoses observing the following classification:

- non-respiratory visits,
- respiratory visits due to upper respiratory symptoms, and
- respiratory visits due to lower respiratory symptoms.

In this case, upper respiratory symptoms included inflammation processes that affected the respiratory tract above the larynx such as pharyngitis, common cold, adenoiditis, sinusitis, tonsilitis and otitis media. Lower respiratory illness included inflammatory processes affecting the larynx, trachea, bronchus or lungs such as bronchitis, pneumonia, broncho-pneumonia, bronchial asthma, acute obstructive bronchitis, acute laryngitis and acute tracheitis. The original data collection separated the children into two age groups: less than 2 years old and children from 2 to 14 years old. For each day, the number of medical visits with each diagnosis was totalled across clinics. Each clinic served an average of 2600 children under age 2, and about 16,000 between ages 3 and 14.

The multiple regression analysis demonstrated a statistically significant association between PM_{10} concentration and medical visits for lower respiratory symptoms in children aged 3 to 15 and in children under age 2. PM_{10} was also associated with medical visits related to upper respiratory symptoms in the older cohort, while ozone was associated with visits related to both lower and upper symptoms in the older cohort. For children under age 2, a $50\mu g/m^3$ change in PM_{10} (about half of the mean concentration during the study period) was generally associated with a 4 to 12 per cent increase in lower respiratory symptoms. For children aged 3 to 15 years, the increases in lower respiratory symptoms were in the range of 3 to 9 per cent for a $50\mu g/m^3$ change in PM_{10}.

Ilabaca et al (1999) analysed data in Santiago on ambient $PM_{2.5}$ and respiratory-related emergency visits to a large paediatric hospital. The study was conducted from February 1995 to August 1996. Besides PM_{10} and $PM_{2.5}$, which were collected at four downtown monitors, data were available for sulphur dioxide, nitrogen dioxide and ozone. The analysis indicated a strong association between both PM_{10} and $PM_{2.5}$ and respiratory visits. During the winter season, a $45\mu g/m^3$ (interquartile) increase in $PM_{2.5}$ was associated with a 2.7 per cent (95 per cent CI = 1.1–4.4 per cent) increase in visits for all respiratory illness, and a 6.7 per cent increase (95 per cent CI = 1.7–12 per cent) in the number of visits for pneumonia. For PM_{10} during the winter months, the interquartile range of $76\mu g/m^3$ was associated with a 2.3 per cent (95 per cent CI = 0.1–4.1 per cent) increase in all respiratory illness, and a 7.7 per cent (95 per cent CI= 2.5–13.2 per cent) increase in pneumonia. Oxides of sulphur and nitrogen were also associated with emergency visits.

The magnitude of effects indicated by these two studies (Ostro et al, 1999; Ilabaca et al, 1999) is within the range of effects reported in studies undertaken in Western nations. The latter studies suggest that a $50\mu g/m^3$ change in PM_{10} is associated with a 4 per cent increase in hospital admissions, a 5 to 20 per cent increase in emergency room visits and a 15 per cent increase in lower respiratory symptoms (Dockery and Pope, 1994). The Ostro et al (1999) estimate of about

1.4 per cent per $10\mu g/m^3$ for clinic visits is within the lower end of the range of 1 to 4 per cent reported by Dockery and Pope (1994). The Ilabaca et al (1999) findings of about 0.5 per cent per $10\mu g/m^3$ are lower than Western studies and may reflect issues of cost and accessibility to hospitals for part of the Santiago population.

Estimating the Quantitative Health Impacts

Basic methodology

Epidemiological studies provide the basis for the selected concentration–response relationships between ambient PM_{10} and several adverse health outcomes used for illustrative purposes in this analysis, including premature mortality, hospital admissions, urgent care visits and respiratory symptoms. We have chosen not to generate estimates for asthma symptoms, acute bronchitis and several other outcomes for which epidemiologic data exist since the baseline incidence in Santiago is unknown. For each of the included health endpoints, a relative risk (RR) estimate is determined from the pooled estimates of the available studies. The RR is the increase in the probability of a given health effect associated with a given increase in exposure. The attributable proportion (A) of health effects from air pollution for the entire population can be calculated as:

1) $A = (RR - 1) / RR$

To calculate the expected cases due to air pollution (E), the following formulation was used:

2) $E = A * B * C * P$

where B= population baseline rate of the given health effect, C = the relevant change in air pollution and P = exposed population for each health effect.
    As an example of these calculations, assume:

- the RR for respiratory symptoms is 1.10 for a $10\mu g/m^3$ change in PM_{10};
- every person in the city is exposed to a PM_{10} concentration of $50\mu g/m^3$ and the projected 'standard' is $20\mu g/m^3$;
- people have an average of ten symptoms per year (prevalence = 10/365 =0.027); and
- there are a million people in this city who are expected to respond to PM_{10} with respiratory symptoms.

Given these assumptions, the attributable risk per $10\mu g/m^3$ can be calculated from equation 1 as 0.09 (= 0.1/1.10). Thus, for this example, roughly 9 per cent of the total number of symptoms in the population can be attributed to a $10\mu g/m^3$ change in PM_{10} (or 0.9 per cent per $\mu g/m^3$). Applying these estimates into equation 2, the cases due to air pollution can be obtained:

$E = (0.009) * (0.027) (30) (1,000,000) (365 \text{ days}) = 2.7$ million extra symptom-days due to air pollution.

For our subsequent assessment, estimates of A, B, C and P are needed. A, the attributable risk, is derived from the assessment of the available epidemiological studies. As different measures of PM are used in the studies, estimates were converted to a PM_{10} equivalent. It was assumed that $PM_{2.5} = 0.5$ of PM_{10}, and that PM_{10} equals PM_{13} or PM_{15}, which are measures often used in Europe. Analysis of the size distribution of PM suggests that there are not many particles, on a weight basis, between PM_{10} and PM_{15} (US Environmental Protection Agency, 1996). B is based on available health statistics or extrapolated from other countries. C is obtained from current monitors in each city and an assumed pollution standard, and P is obtained from census or population data for the cities under study.

Mortality

As indicated above, existing meta-analyses of the time-series studies of acute exposure suggest that, after converting the alternative measures of particulate matter used in the original studies to PM_{10}, the effects on mortality are very consistent (Ostro, 1993; Dockery and Pope, 1994; Schwartz, 1994a). Specifically, the mean effect of a $10\mu g/m^3$ change in PM_{10} implied by these studies is approximately 0.8 per cent, with a range of effects of 0.5 per cent to 1.6 per cent. While the use of daily data and acute exposure has many statistical advantages (eg reducing confounding and exposure measurement error), the quantitative implications are not without uncertainty. For example, there is uncertainty regarding the extent of the prematurity of mortality (ie reduction in life expectancy) resulting from acute exposure. Some of the deaths may be displaced by a few days or weeks. It appears, however, that for many of the deaths, particularly those related to cardiovascular outcomes, the prematurity is much greater and may involve several months or more (Zeger et al, 1999; Schwartz, 2000). Thus, the number of cases of premature mortality can be determined from these studies, but the studies do not provide information on the actual amount of life shortening.

The mortality study conducted in Santiago using PM_{10} (Ostro et al, 1996) provides estimates consistent with those found elsewhere. Specifically, this study generates a central estimate of 0.8 per cent increase in mortality per $10\mu g/m^3$ increase in PM_{10} with a 95 per cent CI = 0.5–0.9 per cent. As indicated above, this estimate is also similar to those found in other Latin American cities. Therefore, for a central estimate, 0.8 per cent was selected. For the low estimate, a coefficient consistent with the lower bound in the Santiago study (Ostro et al, 1996) and the central estimate of a recent study of 20 US cities of 0.5 per cent per $10\mu g/m^3$ (Samet et al, 2000b) was selected.

The high estimate was selected using studies of long term exposure. These studies use a prospective cohort design in which a sample is selected and followed over time in many locations. For example, Dockery et al (1993) published results for a 15-year prospective study based on 8000 individuals in six cities in the US. Pope et al (1995) published results of a seven-year prospective study based on 550,000 individuals in 151 cities in the US. These studies use individual-level data so that other factors that affect mortality can be characterized. Specifically, these studies were able to control for mortality risks associated with differences in body mass, occupational exposures, smoking (present and past), alcohol use, age and gender. Once the effects of individual-level factors are determined, the models examine whether longer term city-wide averages in PM are associated with differences in life expectancy. Both of these studies report a robust and statistically significant association between exposure to PM (usually measured as $PM_{2.5}$) and mortality.

Estimates based on the long term exposure studies are preferable since they include most of the effects of both long and short term exposure and clearly represent a significant reduction in life expectancy. For long term exposure, the estimates from the reanalysis by Krewski et al (2000) of the American Cancer Society (ACS) cohort data originally analysed by Pope et al (1995) were used. The Krewski et al (2000) coefficients were used in preference to those of Pope et al (1995), as the former used the mean rather than median estimates of long term concentrations of $PM_{2.5}$. The mean may better reflect the long term cumulative exposure to PM and is more sensitive to peak concentrations.

Although Krewski et al (2000) also provided estimates based on the Harvard six-cities mortality study (Dockery et al, 1993), only the Krewski analysis of the ACS data was used as it was based on more people and cities (295,000 subjects from 50 cities throughout the US versus 8000 subjects from six Midwest and East Coast cities). The Dockery et al (1993) analysis of the Harvard data, as well as the Krewski et al (2000) reanalysis of these data, generated a larger effect on premature mortality than did the analyses of the ACS cohort.

Based on the estimates derived from the ACS cohort, the estimate of a 4.62 per cent ($\pm$ 1.2) increase in annual mortality per $10\mu g/m^3$ of $PM_{2.5}$ to the population older than age 30 was applied. For PM_{10}, this coefficient was adjusted by the $PM_{2.5}/PM_{10}$ ratio of 0.55, which assumes that only the fine particle share of PM_{10} is toxic. This adjustment was based on the reanalysis of the ACS data set by Pope and others cited in Krewski et al (2000), which shows that for long term exposure, coarse particles (PM_{10}–$PM_{2.5}$) were not associated with mortality. This assumption leads to much lower effects from PM_{10}. Since the original studies only involved adults, the resulting coefficient of 2.54 per cent per $10\mu g/m^3$ is applied to the population above age 21. The baseline annual mortality rate was assumed to equal that reported by Cifuentes et al (2000) of 0.004. Summaries of the coefficients used for mortality and morbidity are provided in Table 10.1.

Morbidity

Dose–response functions and associated relative risks have been developed from studies in the US, Canada, Europe and Latin America for several morbidity endpoints. Below, we detail the estimates that were developed for the risks from

PM on hospital admissions, urgent care visits and respiratory symptoms based on studies of short term exposure.

For many health endpoints, multiple studies were available. To combine the study results into one central estimate and associated confidence intervals, a meta-analytic approach was used. Specifically, the overall effect estimate was developed by weighting each single study estimate by the inverse of the variance of the estimated effect. Following Künzli et al (1999), heterogeneity among the studies was also examined using the Q-test (Petitti, 1994). If the Q-test indicated that the studies were fairly similar, a simple weighting or fixed effects model was used. When significant heterogeneity among the studies was apparent, random effect estimates were used based on the method developed by DerSimonian and Laird (1986). This method adds the variance existing between studies to the reported variance within a given study, thereby changing the study weights. This technique can either raise or lower the central estimate of the effect.

Cardiovascular hospital admissions

There is evidence from studies conducted in several cities of an association between daily changes in PM and changes in hospital admissions for cardiovascular disease. Following Künzli et al (1999), four studies conducted in the European cities of Paris, London, Birmingham and Edinburgh (respectively: Medina et al, 1997; Poloniecki et al, 1997; Wordley et al, 1997; Prescott et al, 1998) were selected to calculate a relative risk of 1.013 (95 per cent CI = 1.007–1.019) per $10\mu g/m^3$. These studies covered all age groups but different time periods between 1987 and 1995, different cardiovascular outcomes and different measures of PM (PM_{10} for Birmingham and Edinburgh and black smoke in the others). Nevertheless, after converting to PM_{10}, the risk estimates were fairly similar across studies.

Three studies from the US and Canada provide additional confirmation of an effect and basis for quantification. Specifically, studies in Detroit (Schwartz and Morris, 1995), Tucson (Schwartz, 1997) and Toronto (Burnett et al, 1997a) were selected. These studies, which all used PM_{10}, provide a joint estimate of 1.008 (95 per cent CI = 1.004–1.011) per $10\mu g/m^3$. These studies also involved different age groups and different measures of cardiovascular disease.

For all studies combined, a fixed effects estimate of 1.009 (95 per cent CI = 1.006–1.013) per $10\mu g/m^3$ was obtained. To develop baseline data on hospital admissions for cardiovascular disease, rates similar to those reported by Kunzli et al (1999) of 0.026 were assumed. Clearly, it would be preferable to use rates generated from data for Santiago.

Respiratory hospital admissions

There is also extensive evidence to indicate that short term changes in PM have impacts on hospital admissions for respiratory disease. Studies are available from both Europe and the US covering various different respiratory endpoints, including all respiratory diseases. From Europe, associations were found in a study combining the results of four cities (London, Amsterdam and Rotterdam and

Paris) using similar protocol from the Air Pollution on Health: a European Approach (APHEA) project (Spix et al, 1998). This study used hospital admissions for all respiratory diseases for the health endpoint, and black smoke for the PM metric. Additional European studies were conducted by Wordley et al (1997) and Prescott et al (1998) for Birmingham and Edinburgh respectively. These studies used specific respiratory disease outcomes and PM_{10}. The Q-test provided evidence of heterogeneity among the studies and the random effects model generated a risk estimate of 1.013 (95 per cent CI = 1.001–1.025) per $10\mu g/m^3$.

Additional estimates are provided by many studies conducted in the US and Canada. Covering a period from 1986 through 1994, the cities include Toronto (Thurston et al, 1994; Burnett et al, 1997b), Detroit (Schwartz, 1994b), Birmingham (Schwartz, 1994c), Minneapolis (Schwartz, 1994d), New Haven and Tacoma (Schwartz, 1995), Spokane (Schwartz, 1996), and Cleveland (Schwartz, 1996). PM_{10} was used in all of these studies and a wide range of ages was included. The Schwartz studies, however, focused on individuals age 65 and above. Heterogeneity was not present among these studies probably because of the similarity in pollution measure and disease coding, and a risk estimate of 1.017 (95 per cent CI = 1.013–1.020) was obtained. Combining the US, Canadian and European studies generated a risk estimate of 1.016 (95 per cent CI= 1.013–1.020) using a random effects model. Baseline incidence for hospital admissions for respiratory disease, derived from Kunzli et al (1999), was 0.013.

Clinic visits

As reviewed above, Ostro et al (1999) found associations between PM_{10} and daily visits to primary healthcare clinics. Associations were found for lower respiratory symptoms in both children under age 2 and 3–15. For children under age 2, a $50\mu g/m^3$ change in PM_{10} was generally associated with a 4 to 12 per cent increase in lower respiratory symptoms, while for children aged 3–15, the change was associated with a 3 to 9 per cent increase. Therefore, it was assumed that a $10\mu g/m^3$ change in PM_{10} is associated with a 1.4 per cent increase in lower respiratory symptoms with a range of 0.7 to 2.1 per cent. The baseline number of urgent care visits for lower respiratory symptoms was 215.4 per day for the eight clinics that served about 12 per cent (n = 153,500) of the population of children in the region. This converts to a baseline incidence rate of 0.0014 per child per day or 0.51 per child per year.

Respiratory symptoms

Several studies provide estimates of the effect of PM on respiratory symptoms. Ostro et al (1993) indicate an association between PM and lower, but not upper, respiratory symptoms among adults in Los Angeles. Using a similar data set, Krupnick et al (1990) reported an association between PM and all symptoms. These studies involved a panel of 300 non-smoking adults followed over a three-month period. PM was measured as sulphates, which are assumed to equal 0.25 of PM_{10}. Using the 1993 study, the results indicate that a $10\mu g/m^3$ change in PM_{10} generates a relative risk of lower respiratory symptoms of 1.07 (95 per

Table 10.1 *Annual health effects in Santiago associated with PM$_{10}$ annual average of 30µg/m^3*

Health endpoint	Reference	% change per 10µg/m^3 (± 95% CI)/	Expected incidence in cases per year		
			Low	Mean	High
Mortality					
Lower bound (all ages):	Samet et al (2000); Ostro et al (1996)	0.5	440		
Central (all ages)	Ostro et al (1996); pooled studies (see text)	0.8		700	
Upper bound (age 30+)	Krewski et al (2000)*	2.54			1300
Hospitalization					
Cardiovascular (all ages)	Pooled studies (see text)	0.9 (0.6–1.3)	3400	5100	7400
Respiratory (all ages)	Pooled studies (see text)	1.6 (1.3–2)	3700	4600	5700
Minor illlness					
Clinic visits (<age 18)	Ostro et al (2000)	1.4 (0.7–2.1)	31,000	63,000	94,000
Lower respiratory symptoms (all ages)	Ostro et al (1993)	7 (2–11)	199,000	696,000	1,090,000

Note: * = coefficient for PM$_{2.5}$ was divided by 0.55 assuming that only the fine particulate share of PM$_{10}$ was associated with mortality from long term exposure.

cent CI = 1.02–1.11). On average, the baseline prevalence of lower respiratory symptoms was 14.24 days per year or 0.039. These results are supported by the findings of Pope et al (1991) and Schwartz et al (1994). Pope et al (1991) reported an association between PM$_{10}$ and the daily reporting of lower respiratory symptoms among a school-based cohort. Schwartz et al (1994) reported an association between PM$_{10}$ and the daily incidence of both coughs and lower respiratory symptoms (defined as two or more symptoms) among a population of schoolchildren. As lower respiratory symptoms appear to be associated with PM$_{10}$ in both children and adults, the coefficient of Ostro et al (1993) was applied to the entire population.

QUANTITATIVE RESULTS

The following estimates for Santiago of health effects of PM$_{10}$ were based on a population of 5 million, a current annual average PM$_{10}$ concentration of 74µg/m^3 and an assumption that 40 per cent of the population is below the age of 21. The relevant change in ambient PM$_{10}$ or the 'target' concentration needs to be determined. Currently, no threshold level for PM$_{10}$, below which no effects are expected to occur, has been identified. There is also little evidence that the slope of the dose–response function diminishes significantly

Table 10.2 *Annual health effects in Santiago associated with* PM_{10} *annual average of* $20\mu g/m^3$

Health endpoint	Reference	% change per $10\mu g/m^3$ ($\pm$ 95% CI)/	Expected incidence in cases per year		
			Low	Mean	High
Mortality					
Lower bound (all ages):	Samet et al (2000); Ostro et al (1996)	0.5	500		
Central (all ages)	Ostro et al (1996); pooled studies (see text)	0.8		900	
Upper bound (age 30+)	Krewski et al, 2000[*]	2.54			1600
Hospitalization					
Cardiovascular (all ages)	Pooled studies (see text)	0.9 (0.6–1.3)	4200	6300	9100
Respiratory (all ages)	Pooled studies (see text)	1.6 (1.3–2)	4600	5600	7000
Minor illness					
Clinic visits (<age 18)	Ostro et al (1999)	1.4 (0.7–2.1)	39,000	77,000	116,000
Lower respiratory symptoms (all ages)	Ostro et al (1993)	7 (2–11)	244,000	854,000	1,340,000

Note: [*] = coefficient for $PM_{2.5}$ was divided by 0.55 assuming that only the fine particulate share of PM_{10} was associated with mortality from long term exposure

at lower concentrations. Most current epidemiological evidence suggests a linear or near-linear concentration–response function indicating a continuum of effects down to the lowest PM levels observed in the study sample. For illustrative purposes, therefore, two different ambient standards were used. The first target concentration used was the ambient standard proposed in 1997 by the US EPA for $PM_{2.5}$ of $15\mu g/m^3$. Assuming a 0.5 ratio between $PM_{2.5}$ and PM_{10} in the US (US Environmental Protection Agency, 1996), this is equivalent to $30\mu g/m^3$ PM_{10}. For sensitivity analysis, the European Union-proposed Stage 2 limit value of $20\mu g/m^3$ PM_{10} was used. Table 10.1 summarizes the quantitative estimates of the current effects of air pollution relating to the standard of $30\mu g/m^3$ PM_{10}, while Table 10.2 summarizes the results using a standard of $20\mu g/m^3$ of PM_{10}.

As indicated by Tables 10.1 and 10.2, substantial health effects in Santiago are associated with current ambient concentrations of PM_{10}. For example, using $30\mu g/m^3$ as a baseline concentration suggests a mean estimate of about 700 cases of premature mortality per year (95 per cent CI = 400–1300) and about 5000 and 4600 extra cases of hospitalization for cardiovascular and respiratory disease, respectively. For less severe outcomes, the mean estimates are 60,000 more clinic visits for children and 700,000 more days with acute symptoms for children and adults relating to air pollution. Assuming a baseline concentration of $20\mu g/m^3$ increases the number of cases of premature mortality to 860 (95 per cent CI = 500–1600) and likewise increases the previous morbidity estimates by about 20 per cent.

CONTROL STRATEGIES

In recent years, several alternative pollution control strategies aimed at reducing PM_{10} concentrations in Santiago have been proposed. The most recent plan proposes several options for controlling PM_{10} and $PM_{2.5}$ from mobile, industrial and residential sources in Santiago (Comisión Nacional de Medio Ambiente, 2001). Specifically, the control strategies under consideration include retiring older public buses and replacing them with low emission buses, upgrading pollution control devices on buses, lowering the sulphur content of diesel fuel, adding emissions standards for diesel trucks, requiring engines to meet recent US standards, improving the quality of the gasoline, reducing emissions related to wood use, reducing emissions from industrial sources, increased street cleaning for dust control and additional paving of streets. Some of these control strategies will be implemented immediately, while others are expected to be phased in over the next several years. If implemented, they should provide significant reductions in PM_{10} concentrations and associated health effects.

NOTE

1   The opinions expressed in this paper are those of the author and do not represent the views or the policies of the California Environmental Protection Agency or the State of California.

REFERENCES

Burnett, R T, Cakmak, S, Brook, J R and Krewski, D (1997a) 'The role of particulate size and chemistry in the association between summertime ambient air pollution and hospitalization for cardiorespiratory diseases' in *Environmental Health Perspectives*, vol 105, pp614–620

Burnett, R T, Brook, J R, Yung, W T, Dales, R E and Krewski, D (1997b) 'Association between ozone and hospitalization for respiratory diseases in 16 Canadian cities' in *Environmental Research*, vol 72, pp24–31

Burnett, R T, Brook, J R, Dann, T, Delocla, C, Philips, O, Calmak, S, Vincent, R, Goldberg, M S and Krewski, D (2000) 'Associations between particulate- and gas-phase components of urban air pollution and daily mortality in eight Canadian cities' in L D Grant (ed) 'PM2000: particulate matter and health' in *Inhalation Toxicology*, vol 12 (suppl 4), pp15–39

Castillejos, M, Borja-Aburto, V H, Dockery, D W, Gold, D R and Loomis, D (2000) 'Airborne coarse particles and mortality' in 'Inhalation toxicology: proceedings of the third colloquium on particulate air pollution and human health, June 1999, Durham, NC' in *Inhalation Toxicology*, vol 12 (suppl 1), pp67–72

Cifuentes, L A, Vega, J, Kopfer, K and Lave, L B (2000) 'Effect of the fine fraction of particulate matter versus the coarse mass and other pollutants on daily mortality in Santiago, Chile' in *Journal of the Air and Waste Management Association*, vol 50, no 8, pp1287–1298

Comisión Nacional de Medio Ambiente (1997) *Plan de Prevención y Descontaminación Atmosférica de la Región Metropolitana*, Santiago, Chile

DerSimonian, R and Laird, N (1986) 'Meta-analysis in clinical trials' in *Controlled Clinical Trials*, vol 7, pp177–188

Dockery, D W, Pope, C A III, Xu, X, Spengler, J D, Ware, J H, Fay, M E, Ferris, B G and Speizer, F E (1993) 'An association between air pollution and mortality in six US cities' in *New England Journal of Medicine*, vol 329, pp1753–1759

Dockery, D W and Pope, C A III (1994) 'Acute respiratory effects of particulate air pollution' in *Annual Review of Public Health*, vol 15, pp107–132

Ilabaca, M, Olaeta, I, Campos, E, Villaire, J, Tellez-Rojo, M M and Romieu, I (1999) 'Association between levels of fine particulate and emergency visits for pneumonia and other respiratory illnesses among children in Santiago, Chile' in *Journal of the Air and Waste Management Association*, vol 49 (9 Spec No), pp154–163

Krewski, D, Burnett, R, Goldberg, M S, Koover, K, Siemiatycki, J, Jerrett, M, Abrahamowicz, M, White, W H et al (2000) 'Reanalysis of the Harvard six cities study and the American Cancer Society study of particulate air pollution and mortality' in *Health Effects Institute* (a special report of the Institute's Particle Epidemiology Reanalysis Project)

Krupnick, A J and Harrington, W (1990) 'Ambient ozone and acute health effects: evidence from daily data' in *Journal of Environmental Economics and Management*, vol 18, pp1–18

Kunzli, N, Kaiser, R, Medina, S, Studnicka, M, Oberfeld, G and Horak, F (1999) 'Health costs due to road traffic-related air pollution, an impact assessment project of Austria, France and Switzerland: air pollution attributable cases', prepared for the Ministerial Conference for Environmental Health

Lippmann, M, Ito, K, Nadas, A and Burnett, R T (2000) 'Association of particulate matter components with daily mortality and morbidity in urban populations' in *Health Effects Institute*, vol 95, pp5–72, discussion pp73–82

Mar, T F, Norris, G A, Koenig, J Q and Larson, T V (2000) 'Associations between air pollution and mortality in Phoenix, 1995–1997' in *Environment Health Perspectives*, vol 108, no 4, pp347–353

Medina, S, Le Tertre, A, Quenel, P, Le Moullec, Y, Lameloise, P, Guzzo, J C, Festy, B, Ferry, R and Dab, W (1997) 'Air pollution and doctors' house calls: results from the ERPURS system for monitoring the effects of air pollution on public health in Greater Paris, France, 1991–1995' in *Environmental Research*, vol 75, pp73–84

Ostro, B D (1993) 'The association of air pollution and mortality: examining the case for inference' in *Archives of Environmental Health*, vol 48, no 5, pp336–342

Ostro, B D, Lipsett, M J, Mann, J K, Krupnick, A and Harrington, W (1993) 'Air pollution and respiratory morbidity among adults in southern California' in *American Journal of Epidemiology*, vol 137, no 7, pp691–700

Ostro, B D, Sanchez, J M, Aranda, C and Eskeland, G S (1996) 'Air pollution and mortality: results from a study in Santiago, Chile' in *Journal of Exposure Analysis and Environmental Epidemiology*, vol 6, pp97–114

Ostro, B D, Eskeland, G S, Sanchez, J M and Feyzioglu, T (1999) 'Air pollution and health effects: a study of medical visits among children in Santiago, Chile' in *Environment Health Perspectives*, vol 107, pp69–73

Petitti, D B (1994) *Meta-analysis, Decision Analysis and Cost Effectiveness Analysis: Methods for Quantitative Synthesis in Medicine*, Oxford University Press, New York/Oxford

Poloniecki, J D, Atkinson, R W, de Leon, A P and Anderson, H R (1997) 'Daily time series for cardiovascular hospital admissions and previous day's air pollution in London, UK' in *Occupational Environmental Medicine*, vol 54, pp535–540

Pope, C A III, Dockery, D W, Spenglerf, J and Raizenne, M E (1991) 'Respiratory health and PM[10] pollution – a daily time series analysis' in *American Review of Respiratory Diseases*, vol 144, pp668–674

Pope, C A III, Thun, M J, Namboodiri, M M, Dockery, D W, Evans, J S, Speizer, F E and Heath, C W Jr (1995) 'Particulate air pollution as a predictor of mortality in a prospective study of US adults' in *American Journal of Respiratory and Critical Care Medicine*, vol 151, pp669–674

Prescott, G J, Cohen, G R, Elton, R A, Fowkes, F G and Agius, R M (1998) 'Urban air pollution and cardiopulmonary ill health: a 14.5 year time series study' in *Occupational and Environmental Medicine*, vol 55, pp697–704

Saldiva, P H N and Bohm, G M (1995) 'Air pollution and mortality in Sao Paulo, Brazil', unpublished paper, Faculty of Medicine, University of Sao Paulo, Sao Paulo, pp1–19

Samet, J M, Dominici, F, Curriero, F C, Coursac, I and Zeger, S L (2000) 'Fine particulate air pollution and mortality in 20 US cities, 1987–1994' in *New England Journal of Medicine*, vol 343, no 24, pp1742–1749

Schwartz, J (1994a) 'Air pollution and daily mortality: a review and meta-analysis' in *Environmental Research*, vol 64, pp36–52

Schwartz, J (1994b) 'Air pollution and hospital admissions for the elderly in Detroit, Michigan' in *American Journal of Respiratory and Critical Care Medicine*, vol 150, no 3, pp648–655

Schwartz, J (1994c) 'Air pollution and hospital admissions for the elderly in Birmingham, Alabama' in *American Journal of Epidemiology*, vol 139, pp589–598

Schwartz, J (1994d) 'PM[10], ozone, and hospital admissions for the elderly in Minneapolis-St Paul, Minnesota' in *Archives of Environmental Health*, vol 49, no 5, pp366–374

Schwartz, J (1995) 'Short term fluctuations in air pollution and hospital admissions of the elderly for respiratory disease' in *Thorax*, vol 50, pp531–538

Schwartz, J (1996) 'Air pollution and hospital admissions for respiratory disease' in *Epidemiology*, vol 7, pp20–28

Schwartz, J (1997) 'Air pollution and hospital admissions for cardiovascular disease in Tucson' in *Epidemiology*, vol 8, pp371–377

Schwartz, J (2000) 'Harvesting and long term exposure effects in the relationship between air pollution and mortality' in *American Journal of Epidemiology*, vol 151, pp440–448

Schwartz, J, Dockery, D W, Neas, L M, Wypij, D, Ware, J H, Spengler, J D, Koutrakis, P, Speizer, F E and Ferris, B G Jr (1994) 'Acute effects of summer air pollution on respiratory symptom reporting in children' in *American Journal of Respiratory and Critical Care Medicine*, vol 150 (5 Pt 1), pp1234–1242

Schwartz, J and Morris, R (1995) 'Air pollution and hospital admissions for cardiovascular disease in Detroit, Michigan' in *American Journal of Epidemiology*, vol 142, no 1, pp23–25

Schwartz, J, Dockery, D W and Neas, L M (1996) 'Is daily mortality associated with specifically with fine particles?' in *Journal of the Air & Waste Management Association*, vol 46, pp927–939

Spix, C, Anderson, H R, Schwartz, J, Vigotti, M A, LeTertre, A, Vonk, J M, Touloumi, G, Balducci, F, Piekarski, T, Bacharova, L, Tobias, A, Ponka, A and Katsouyanni, K

(1998) 'Short term effects of air pollution on hospital admissions of respiratory diseases in Europe: a quantitative summary of APHEA study results' in *Archives of Environmental Health*, vol 53, pp54–64

Thurston, G D, Ito, K, Hayes, C G, Bates, D V and Lippmann, M (1994) 'Respiratory hospital admissions and summertime haze air pollution in Toronto, Ontario: consideration of the role of acid aerosols' in *Environmental Research*, vol 65, pp271–290

US Environmental Protection Agency (1996) *Air Quality Criteria for Particulate Matter*, EPA/600/P-95/001cF, Office of Research and Development

Wordley, J, Walters, S and Ayres, J G (1997) 'Short term variations in hospital admissions and mortality and particulate air pollution' in *Occupational and Environmental Medicine*, vol 54, no 2, pp108–116

Zeger, S L, Dominici, F and Samet, J (1999) 'Harvesting-resistant estimates of air pollution effects on mortality' in *Epidemiology*, vol 10, no 2, pp171–175

11

Air Quality and Health in Greater Johannesburg

Angela Mathee and Yasmin von Schirnding

ABSTRACT

The city of Johannesburg is one of the fastest growing on the African continent. With sprawling squatter and informal settlements, rapid industrialization and a weak public transport system, Johannesburg is typical of many cities in developing countries. In this chapter we draw attention to the fact that urban air pollution is a major public health concern in Johannesburg. As is so frequently the case in many cities throughout the world, the potential for effectively addressing the air pollution situation in Johannesburg is constrained by limited resources, capacity for essential research and monitoring and management capability overall.

Here we describe the overall air quality situation (using the available research and monitoring data) and discuss the implications for public health in Johannesburg, with particular attention to high risk settings and the roles of poverty and former apartheid-based planning and policies in determining the groups at greatest risk of exposure. Also addressed in this chapter are the national and local programmes implemented to reduce air pollution, and some of the weaknesses of the current policies and legislative framework. Recommendations are made for long and shorter term improvements and actions to reduce public exposure to excessive levels of key air pollutants.

INTRODUCTION

In this chapter the conditions and processes that have implications for air quality and health in the city of Johannesburg are outlined. Available information from surveillance programmes and various studies is used to describe the air quality and health situation, and a selection of local, national and international policy and programme options to improve air quality in Johannesburg are outlined.

Johannesburg is one of the fastest growing urban areas on the African continent (Beall, 2000). The city houses around 3 million people, but forms part of an urban agglomeration of around 8 million people. Johannesburg is considered to be the economic heartland of South Africa. In recent years the city's economy has been based mainly on manufacturing, industrial and financial services, and whilst no longer the main focus of the economy, primary mining continues in the nearby West Rand. Several mine tailings dumps located mainly in the south of the city are currently being reprocessed. These and other activities continue to attract large numbers of people to Johannesburg. Economic growth rates, though, have lagged behind population growth, resulting in increased unemployment and poverty in the city (Beall, 2000).

Johannesburg is located around a series of low, rocky ridges at an altitude of 1500–1800m above sea level. The climate is temperate, with about eight hours of sunlight per day and an average temperature of 22.4°C. Winters are cold and dry, with rainfall averaging about 710mm per annum, mainly in the form of late afternoon summer electrical storms. The climate is unfavourable for the dispersion of air pollution, and inversion conditions occur frequently, especially during the winter.

There are three main scenarios of exposure to elevated levels of air pollution in Johannesburg. The first is the sprawling and crowded townships and informal settlements in and around the city, associated with a process of rapid, unplanned urbanization which has occurred in recent decades. The townships of Soweto and Alexandra, and their associated informal settlements (see Figure 11.1), are two examples of settings in which serious air pollution problems have occurred. The second scenario of exposure is the emission of various pollutants from industrial sites, which have been associated with inadequate control measures and the weak enforcement of existing legislation. The third major area of concern is emissions from vehicles (which are, on average, older than those in developed countries) and poor public transport and traffic management systems.

Little detailed information is available on the extent of the impact of air pollution in Johannesburg on the health of its population. However, there is an accumulating body of evidence from various parts of South Africa suggesting that urban air pollution is associated with an increased prevalence of respiratory symptoms in certain groups of young children, including acute respiratory infections (ARIs), a leading cause of death in young children under the age of five years (von Schirnding et al, 1991a). A study undertaken in the early 1990s revealed that the mortality rate for ARI amongst 'coloured' infants was around 980 per 100,000, which was about ten times higher than the rate for white infants. While death rates from pneumonia in all population groups have shown a substantial decline over the past two decades, in some urban areas of South Africa there is nevertheless evidence that deaths from ARI are now more significant than those from diarrhoea (von Schirnding et al, 1991b). In the following sections available information from surveillance programmes and

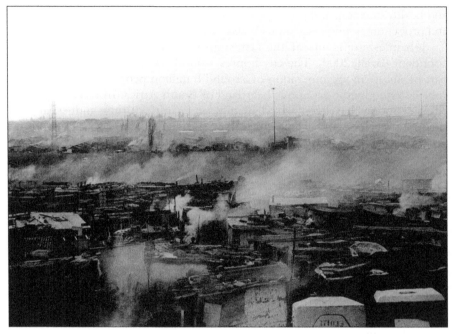

Figure 11.1 *Smoke from winter fires in the township of Alexandra, Johannesburg*

studies is used to describe the air pollution situation and health implications in key Johannesburg settings.

URBANIZATION

The unplanned movement of large numbers of people into Johannesburg has resulted in the formation of sprawling squatter and informal settlements on the city periphery and smaller sites in inner city areas. Informal and squatter settlements are currently estimated to house around 20 per cent of the city population (approximately 640,000 people). In these settlements, as well as in many urban townships originally designed (under the apartheid system) to house black people, large proportions of households do not have access to (or cannot afford to use) electricity, and instead rely on fuels such as coal, wood and kerosene for domestic purposes. Under these conditions, indoor air pollution levels, as well as ambient air pollution levels, may exceed international health standards, especially during the cold winter months (see Figure 11.1).

Under apartheid, the township of Soweto was created to house the urban black population serving Johannesburg. Associated with waves of urbanization and forced removals from other sites in Johannesburg, the Soweto population rapidly grew to the current estimate of 1 million, a large proportion of whom live in informal settlements or informal backyard dwellings. Since its inception, Soweto has been characterized by poor housing and environmental conditions, among which has been the use of coal, wood and kerosene for cooking and the heating of water and space, resulting in high levels of ambient and indoor air pollution.

The birth-to-ten study

In 1990, the collaborative birth-to-ten (BTT) research project was initiated with the broad aim of assessing the environmental, economic, psycho-social and biological determinants of health, development and wellbeing amongst a cohort of 3275 children from birth to the age of ten years in Soweto and parts of Johannesburg. All singleton births to women who were permanent residents of Johannesburg and Soweto during a seven-week period between April and June 1990 were included in the study (Yach et al, 1991). Aspects investigated included pre-natal risk factors, childhood mortality and morbidity, environmental risk factors in the home and broader living environment, and health status (including the prevalence of diarrhoeal disease and ARIs, and growth and psychological development).

Questionnaires related to a wide range of concerns were administered to the entire cohort ante-natally, as well as annually or biennially, for the duration of the study. At the time of birth, cord blood samples were collected for analysis of lead concentrations. Information was also collected through air pollution monitoring programmes implemented in association with various organizations – related to sulphur dioxide (SO_2), nitrogen oxides (NO_x), ozone (O_3), fine particulate mass and various meteorological parameters measured on a continuous basis at a stationary site – as well as data relating to particulate pollution collected at nine sites in Soweto.

Specific areas of research interest were also investigated in relation to selected sub-cohorts under the broad umbrella of the BTT project. For example, air pollution and respiratory health was the focus of a nested longitudinal sub-study of 328 BTT children drawn from low lying and high lying Soweto suburbs, thought to be associated with high and low levels of air pollution respectively (von Schirnding and Mokoetle, 1993). Over a period of around one year a structured questionnaire aimed at obtaining information related to housing factors, fuel use patterns, respondents' perceptions of the health of the child, ill-health symptoms using a two-week recall period and major illnesses since birth was administered on a monthly basis to the caretakers of the sub-study children. Health diaries were left at the homes of children in order that daily ill-health symptoms experienced by the study child could be recorded. Stationary indoor monitoring was undertaken in a sample of the homes of study children from high and low lying areas.

Findings of birth-to-ten air pollution monitoring programmes

The BTT PM_{10} ambient air monitoring programme showed that for the duration of the project, winter levels usually exceeded South African guideline values. For example, during 1999, PM_{10} levels equalling $150\mu g/m^3$ and $50\mu g/m^3$ were measured during winter and summer respectively (24-hour sampling undertaken

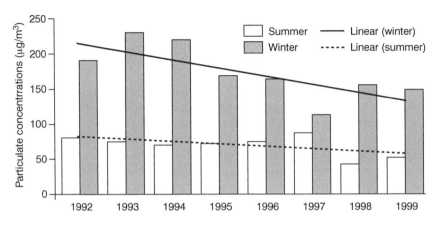

Source: Annegarn and Sithole, 1999

Figure 11.2 *Airborne particulate concentrations in Soweto, 1992–1999*

every sixth day and averaged over a season of three months). Looking at trends over the first nine years of air quality monitoring for the project, an overall decrease in PM_{10} levels (an average annual decrement of $12\mu g/m^3$) was noted (see Figure 11.2). Whilst no specific intervention could be associated with the improvement observed, environmental upliftment programmes implemented during this period included improvements in electricity supply, paving of roads, improved industrial control measures and grassing of mine dumps (Annegarn and Sithole, 1999).

Health aspects of the birth-to-ten study

The results for the full BTT cohort showed that 50 per cent of children who lived in homes with an open fire experienced respiratory related symptoms such as sneezing or a runny/stuffy nose, compared to 24 per cent of children who lived in homes without open fires. Thirty-one per cent of caretakers who perceived that air pollution was a problem reported that their children had sneezing and runny/stuffy nose symptoms in the previous two weeks, compared to 23 per cent who did not perceive air pollution to be a problem. Pets in the home was also a risk factor, with 29 per cent of people with pets in the home having children who had symptoms relating to sneezing and a runny/stuffy nose compared with 21 per cent of children who lived in homes without pets. Five per cent of children who lived in homes with smokers experienced difficulty breathing and fever, compared with 2 per cent of children who lived in homes without smokers.

Regarding the sub-study of 328 children, results indicated that whilst 91 per cent of dwellings were supplied with electricity, the use of a two-week recall period to ascertain recent energy use patterns showed that households used electricity as their main cooking fuel in only 67 per cent of dwellings, whilst coal and paraffin (kerosene) had been the principal fuel used in 25 per cent and 8 per cent of dwellings respectively. In terms of space heating, 52 per cent had used mainly electricity, while 43 per cent and 5 per cent respectively had used mainly coal and paraffin. More than half (55 per cent) of respondents reported that the house became smoky when the fire was burning. Sixty-one per cent of respondents reported that a family member regularly smoked, and in 11 per cent of dwellings one or more people smoked more than 20 cigarettes each day. In 37 per cent of dwellings, the study child was reported to usually be in the kitchen when cooking was undertaken.

In terms of health, 54 per cent of respondents reported that children had experienced colds and chest illness with high frequency since birth. Runny noses (53 per cent), sneezing (38 per cent) and a productive cough (28 per cent) were amongst the most frequently reported ill-health symptoms using a two week recall period. Ear infections (8 per cent), bronchitis/bronchiolitis (5 per cent), pneumonia (4 per cent) and allergies (4 per cent) were amongst the most frequently reported health problems diagnosed by a doctor since the birth of the child. By around 14 months of age, 4 per cent of children in the sub-study had been admitted to hospital for a chest illness.

Amongst the environmental risk factors identified for respiratory ill-health were living in a low lying (relatively 'polluted') area of Soweto (associated with elevated reporting of wheezing using a two-week recall period), living in homes with leaks or water damage (higher levels of wheezing and fever), usually being in the kitchen during cooking periods (more likely to be perceived as unhealthy compared to other children of a similar age, and higher levels of colds and chest illness since birth), and living in homes where animals were kept or where cockroaches were a problem.

Other metropolitan areas

Additional evidence of respiratory health effects associated with air pollution comes from a survey of some of the major metropolitan areas in South Africa, which indicated that domestic fuel combustion (coal for example) was associated with excess respiratory symptoms in young children (von Schirnding et al, 1991b). For example, 29 per cent of children under five years were reported to have experienced coughing and breathing problems in a two-week recall period. Multiple logistic regression analyses revealed that, among other factors, the absence of electricity was independently associated with respiratory symptoms.

Sulphur dioxide

The use of coal and wood for domestic purposes in informal dwellings is of concern also in relation to exposure to SO_2. During 1999, as part of a partnership between the Greater Johannesburg Metropolitan Council, the Council for Scientific and Industrial Research and the Swedish Environmental Research Institute, levels of SO_2 and nitrogen dioxide (NO_2) were monitored at over 200 sites in Johannesburg using passive samplers over a period of one winter month. The results indicated a city-wide mean SO_2 level of $30\mu g/m^3$, with the minimum and maximum levels respectively equalling 14 and $70\mu g/m^3$.

The highest levels of SO_2 were recorded in the vicinity of dense and sprawling townships and informal settlements, such as those in Soweto and Alexandra, where frequent use is made of solid fuels such as coal and wood (GJMC/IVL/CSIR, 1999).

INDUSTRIALIZATION

Areas zoned for industrial use are located across and in close proximity to the city, especially in the southern parts, and mining operations in and around the city are ongoing. The Vaal Triangle for example, which is located around 40km from the centre of the city of Johannesburg, houses petrochemical, chemical, brick, tile, steel and numerous other operations. In addition, more than 1 million people who use coal for domestic purposes live in the vicinity.

The Vaal Triangle air pollution and health study

An air pollution and health study involving 11,000 schoolchildren aged 8 to 12 years was undertaken in the Vaal Triangle over the period 1990 to 1993 in response to ongoing complaints about perceived health impacts resulting from industrial emissions in the area.

The results of the air monitoring component of the Vaal Triangle study showed that levels of SO_2 and O_3 exceeded the reference values of the US National Ambient Air Quality Standards around 5 per cent and 1 per cent of the time respectively, whilst levels of carbon monoxide (CO) and oxides of nitrogen were within the recommended limits throughout the study period. In terms of particulate matter (PM), an annual average of $180\mu g/m^3$ of total suspended particulate matter (TSP) was measured for the study period, which was more than double the US EPA standard at the time. Personal monitoring was undertaken amongst 124 children from no-smoking homes in a relatively unpolluted site. The results showed that 60 per cent of children were exposed to TSP levels above US EPA standards. Measurements of personal exposures amongst 45 children from a coal-burning township, on the other hand, showed that 100 per cent of measurements exceeded EPA standards. Whilst summer exposures were lower than those measured during winter, TSP exceedances occurred throughout the year. Exposures were lower amongst children living in electrified dwellings. Overall, the risk factors for the highest levels of exposure to TSP were season (winter), the use of coal for domestic purposes, the use of braziers rather than stoves, and gender (boys tended to have higher exposures relative to girls) (Terblanche, 1998). An inventory of the sources of PM indicated that despite a higher level of emission of PM from industrial origin, in terms of human exposure and ill-health outcomes, particulates from household coal burning were the greatest risk factor. An air characterization study indicated that up to 70 per cent of the particulate pollution in the area resulted from coal burning and dust, whilst the remainder was linked to industrial activities and motor vehicles (Van Nierop and Annegarn, 1993).

Health aspects of the Vaal Triangle study

In terms of health, high levels of respiratory illness were documented throughout the study period. In general, the prevalence of upper respiratory tract infections annually was 65 per cent, while the level for lower respiratory illness was 29 per cent. Children who had been living in the Vaal Triangle since birth had a significantly elevated prevalence of lower respiratory illnesses compared to children who had lived there from the age of five years. In coal burning townships, amongst children from homes in which electricity was used, the risk of developing upper respiratory symptoms was nine times lower than amongst their counterparts living in coal using dwellings. The use of kerosene also conferred health benefits over the use of coal (Terblanche, 1998).

In a case-control component of the longitudinal study, respiratory illness rates amongst 4713 Vaal Triangle children were compared with those in 2433 children in a less polluted region (Klerksdorp) during the summer of 1992. The findings showed an elevation of 21 to 103 per cent in the risk of developing respiratory illness in the Vaal Triangle compared to Klerksdorp (Terblanche, 1998).

The Vaal Triangle researchers concluded that air pollution in the area, especially PM, significantly exceeded international guideline values at the time, and placed the health of approximately 2 million people in the region at risk. Local children especially had an elevated risk of respiratory ill-health. The use of coal in domestic settings was determined to be the most important risk factor for respiratory ill-health, followed by industrial and natural sources. Despite the strong evidence of health impacts associated with elevated levels of particulate air pollution in the area, abatement action was slow to emerge.

TRANSPORT AND TRAFFIC

Land use planning associated with the apartheid era has resulted in the location of black residential townships well away from sites of work, leading to the need for extended daily commuting journeys in the city. The public transport system in Johannesburg is weak, with a heavy reliance on road-based, privately owned vehicles. Rail systems and bus routes service only parts of the city. The weakness of the public transport system has spawned a burgeoning, informal mini-bus taxi industry, which covers large cross-sections of the city but has been marked to a significant degree by badly tuned vehicles in a state of disrepair, and is associated also with elevated traffic accidents and mortality and injury rates.

A number of routine air quality monitoring programmes covering varying periods and pollutants have been in place in Johannesburg since the 1950s, whilst special studies have been undertaken from time to time. Pollutants monitored include methane, non-methane hydrocarbons, NO_x, NO_2, O_3, CO, SO_2, PM and lead. However, monitoring, analysis and use of the data collected have not always been optimal in terms of assessment of the implications for, and protection of, public health. For example, monitoring stations are frequently placed at sites of little relevance to health (such as alongside main roads or on top of multi-storey buildings).

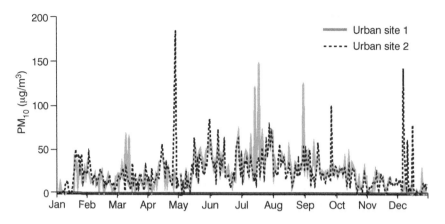

Figure 11.3 *Mean daily PM₁₀ levels in Johannesburg, 2000*

As can be seen from Figure 11.3, the results of the 1999 PM_{10} monitoring programme (relatively less influenced by location) at two Johannesburg inner city sites indicated that levels were slightly elevated during winter relative to summer, and that peaks as high as $181\mu g/m^3$ were measured over a 24-hour period from time to time. Decreases in levels of PM_{10} and $PM_{2.5}$ were noted in a study undertaken in the Johannesburg suburb of Randburg over a four-year period from 1996 (Engelbrecht and Swanepoel, 2000).

In respect of NO_2, results from the GJMC/CSIR/IVL study showed that the highest levels were recorded around the central Johannesburg business district and in the Sandton area, where development has been particularly rapid during recent years, resulting also in an increased daily influx of motor vehicles and high levels of traffic congestion. The study indicated a city-wide NO_2 mean for the month of $39\mu g/m^3$, with the minimum and maximum levels equalling 15 and $62\mu g/m^3$ respectively. However, in parts of the city where traffic was dense, the mean NO_2 level was as high as $48\mu g/m^3$ (GJMC/CSIR/IVL, 1999).

Lead in the environment

The South African petrol lead level has been reduced in stages from an initial concentration of 0.836g/litre in the 1980s to the current maximum permissible concentration of 0.4g/litre, and the introduction in 1996 of unleaded petrol. However, the transition to using unleaded petrol is expected to be relatively slow because of the slow replacement of ageing vehicles. By 1998, despite a tax differential at the time to encourage its use, only 10–15 per cent of petrol sales were of the unleaded variety. The removal of lead from petrol will also pave the way for the mandatory installation of catalytic converters in new vehicles, which is expected to bring about considerable improvements in exhaust emissions.

In the past, annual average air lead levels recorded at major urban centres in South Africa frequently exceeded the World Health Organization (WHO) guideline of $0.5\mu g/m^3$. In Johannesburg, for example, annual air lead levels recorded in 1992, 1994 and 1996 respectively equalled 0.53, 0.50 and $0.86\mu g/m^3$.

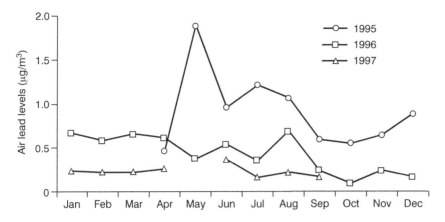

Figure 11.4 *Monthly air lead levels in Johannesburg, 1995–1997*

Since 1996, air lead levels in Johannesburg (see Figure 11.4), as well as in other major cities in the country, appear to have been decreasing (www.ngo.grida.no/soesa/nsoer/indicatr). However, in certain parts of the city fallout leading to high soil lead concentrations remains a concern. In a recent preliminary investigation of the lead content of soil from the playgrounds of nine Johannesburg inner city schools, soil lead concentrations ranged up to 767μg/g, with four schools having levels exceeding 80μg/g.

Blood lead levels among Johannesburg school children and newborns

In 1995, the former Johannesburg City Council, in conjunction with the South African Medical Research Council, undertook a study of the blood lead distribution amongst grade one children attending selected schools in the Johannesburg inner city, as well as in the low income suburbs of Westbury and Newclare and the township of Alexandra. This study indicated that blood lead levels of 433 first grade children ranged from 6 to 26 micrograms per decilitre (μg/dl), with the mean level equalling 12μg/dl. Blood lead levels in 78 per cent of the children exceeded the international action level of 10μg/dl (Mathee et al, 1996). Children with high blood lead levels were perceived to perform poorly at school and were considered to be over-active compared to other children. In various studies of the epidemiology of childhood lead exposure in the Cape peninsula, elevated blood lead levels were associated with attending schools in close proximity to busy roads (von Schirnding and Fuggle, 1996; von Schirnding et al, 1991c).

Under the umbrella of the BTT project, a cross-sectional, analytical study of cord blood lead levels and associated risk factors was conducted amongst Soweto newborns. Umbilical cord blood samples were collected at the time of birth, and information related to social and environmental factors was obtained through the administration of questionnaires ante-natally, while additional data were collected from birth records at the time of delivery. Lead levels were measured in cord blood samples taken from 881 newborns. Structured questionnaires administered ante-natally were used to obtain information related to a wide range of socio-environmental factors, including maternal and paternal educational status, economic status, marital status, home language, housing quality, the presence of dust, crowding, fuel usage practices, transport use, the main water source, tobacco use and alcohol consumption. Further information related to, for example, the sex of the baby, birth weight, head circumference, length, gestational age, Apgar scores[1] and the presence of congenital abnormalities were obtained from birth records at the time of delivery.

The blood lead distribution ranged from 2 to 20μg/dl, with the mean level equalling 5.9μg/dl. A number of social and environmental factors were significantly related to cord blood lead levels, including for example levels of crowding, the presence of a separate kitchen for cooking purposes only, and the time of the work-to-home journey. In addition, borderline significance was shown for the type of transport used. Raised cord blood lead levels were associated with the use of public transport as opposed to transport modes such as walking and the use of a private vehicle. A significant relationship was determined with maternal work status, and blood lead levels were also significantly associated with maternal age and the presence of congenital abnormalities (Mathee, 1995).

PROGRAMMES AND POLICIES

South Africa will continue to experience the effects of rapid urbanization and industrialization, as well as transportation and urban traffic, into the foreseeable future, and will experience the environmental problems of both a highly industrialized economy and a developing country. Growth rates are highest in informal settlements in and around cities, and therefore increases in the proportion of the population who are housed informally are likely to continue. With inappropriately planned development and inadequately managed urbanization, air quality could deteriorate further in some areas, particularly if mass electrification programmes in the urban townships are undermined by poverty and there is ongoing use of fossil fuels, particularly lower grade coal. Domestic air pollution therefore must continue to feature on the agenda of the city of Johannesburg, together with industrial and particularly vehicle pollution control.

The longer term solution to the pollution problems in the townships is socio-economic upliftment and the provision of adequate housing and affordable, low cost electricity. In this regard, as part of a national programme of electrification, around 450,000 households have been provided with electricity annually in South Africa since the early 1990s. Initially, the national electrification programme was expected to dramatically reduce indoor and ambient air pollution and improve community respiratory health status. Evaluations, however, have indicated that, years after the provision of electricity, households continue to use coal, wood and other polluting fuels for cooking and space heating. Nonetheless, despite an incomplete transition to the use of electricity, electrification programmes do confer a significant improvement in indoor, and consequently ambient, air quality, as illustrated by a recent comparative study of levels of respirable PM in electrified and un-electrified dwellings (Mathee et al, 2001). Investigations have pointed to poverty and culture as some of the key factors undermining expected air quality and health improvements associated with electrification programmes (Department of Minerals and Energy, 1996).

In the shorter term, public education campaigns are needed to make communities aware of the links between air pollution and ill-health symptoms, and of ways to reduce exposure to indoor air pollution. Research and development into the use of cleaner, energy-efficient low smoke stoves and cleaner low smoke fuels, as well as research into alternative energy technologies, should be continued, involving communities and all stakeholders in devising solutions that are appropriate and acceptable to communities.

Even though the epidemiological studies conducted to date have not pinpointed particular industries in need of improved control measures, it is clear that industrial emissions contribute to worsened air quality and that both scheduled and non-scheduled processes need to be better controlled in South Africa in the future. Increased attention will need to be given to the use of cleaner technologies and alternative sources of energy.

South Africa needs to move quickly towards an integrated pollution control policy, which will protect the total environment from all sources of pollution. Whilst public discussion in this regard is currently under way, air pollution continues to be governed by the Atmospheric Pollution Prevention Control Act 45 of 1965, which has not undergone any major changes since its initial promulgation. The law makes provision for controlling emissions from scheduled processes, which are the main industrial processes such as power stations, metallurgical and chemical processes and others. It is based on the 'best practicable means' philosophy, which makes provision for a flexible approach to air pollution control based on 'doing one's best' within current economic means, but improving as circumstances change. No set standards for air pollution exist that are enforceable by law. Those guideline values that have been developed are applied to the more general pollutants such as SO_2, NO_2, O_3 and others. Air quality standards based on levels required to protect the most vulnerable need to be introduced and enforced. Emission standards need to be reviewed, and programmes introduced for upgrading existing equipment as needed. Additional research into the occurrence of air pollution and on control and abatement measures is needed, as well as localized epidemiological studies to detect health problems in high risk communities.

The best practicable means philosophy is dependant upon regular inspections and is nearly impossible to monitor and enforce, given its inherent subjectivity and the current air pollution inspectorate for the country (which numbers less than ten inspectors). An improvement on the current system would be what is termed the 'best practicable environmental option', which ensures that the best option for the environment is chosen, at an acceptable cost. An integrated pollution control policy for the country would not only ensure that all aspects of the environment are considered in an integrated way, rather than in the current compartmentalized fashion, but would also be able to make more efficient use of different cadres of inspectors, including environmental health officers, to control and monitor pollution. Whatever system is chosen, it is clear that the wide ranging discretionary powers currently given to the chief air pollution control officer for the country will need to be revised. Communities will also need to become more involved in policy development and environmental monitoring programmes.

Appropriate economic incentives and disincentives also need to be devised, including the possibility of a tax on emissions, which could be used as a fund for environmental improvement similar to taxes on tobacco. The 'polluter pays' principle needs to be firmly enshrined. Revised legislation needs to make provision for more stringent fines for polluters. More control needs to be given to local authorities where capacity exists to control and monitor pollution, and uniform regulations developed to control more effectively dust, smoke and odours (the control of smoke from smaller and non-scheduled industries is currently delegated to local authorities).

Overall, in order to ensure sustainable development there will be a need to introduce mass-based education and promotion programmes aimed at changes in lifestyles, coupled with the use of economic incentive measures, integrated environmental management procedures and better land use planning, in addition to the implementation of improved technological air pollution control measures and tougher legislation. Of critical importance is the education of women, which would empower them and enable them to play a more significant role in the overall process of development, and in particular, to help address the problem of domestic air pollution.

International developments have also been critical for improvements in urban environmental quality in general. The United Nations Conference on Environment and Development (the so-called 'Earth Summit') and Agenda 21 (in 1992) raised the profile of the environment and health in planning and decision-making in South Africa and the world. The recent World Summit on Sustainable Development in Johannesburg in 2002 focused attention on the city and the state of its environment: hopefully this will lead to increased efforts to improve air quality in the years to come, leading to associated impacts on health.

ACKNOWLEDGEMENTS

The authors gratefully acknowledge the generous contributions of the following individuals in the preparation of this chapter: Gideon Slabbert, Michael Clark, Harold Annegarn, Jabu Sithole, Corrie Bezuidenhout and Andre Swart.

NOTE

1   Apgar: named for the anaesthetist who originated the system (Virginia Apgar), this is a test commonly carried out on newborns. It gives a score out of ten based on certain characteristics (colour, heartbeat, response to stimulus, muscle tone and breathing). The score provides an indication of the baby's state of health at birth.

REFERENCES

Annegarn, H J and Sithole, J S (1999) *Soweto Air Monitoring: Project SAM – Trend Analysis of Particulate Pollution for the period 1992–1999*, AER99.163 S SAM, Report to the Department of Environmental Affairs and Tourism South Africa, Annegarn Environmental Research, Johannesburg

Beall, J, Crankshaw, O and Parnell, S (2000) 'Local government, poverty reduction and inequality in Johannesburg' in *Environment and Urbanization*, vol 12, pp107–122

Department of Minerals and Energy (1996) *Energy in South Africa – Revision 1*, Department of Minerals and Energy, Pretoria

Engelbrecht, J and Swanepoel, L (2000) *Four Consecutive Years of TSP, PM[10] and PM[2.5] Integrated Aerosol Monitoring at Mintek in Randburg*, paper presented at the Conference of the National Association for Clean Air, Hartebeespoort, South Africa, 14–15 September

GJMC/IVL/CSIR (1999) *Draft Report – Mapping of Air Pollution Levels in Johannesburg, 1999*

Mathee, A (1995) *Cord Blood Lead Levels and Associated Risk Factors in Greater Johannesburg, South Africa*, MSc Thesis, London School of Hygiene and Tropical Medicine, London

Mathee, A, von Schirnding, Y E R, Ismail, A and Huntley, R (1996) 'Surveys of blood lead burdens among school children and newborns in Greater Johannesburg' in *Urbanisation and Health Newsletter*, vol 29, pp43–49

Mathee, A, Rollin, H, Bruce, N and Levin, J (2001) *Household Energy and Health: Report on a South African Feasibility Study*, preliminary research report prepared for the World Health Organization, South African Medical Research Council, Cape Town

Terblanche, P (1998) *Vaal Triangle Air Pollution Health Study: Bibliography, Summary of Key Findings and Recommendations*, South African Medical Research Council, Cape Town

Van Nierop, P S and Annegarn, H J (1993) *Particulate Source Inventory for the Vaal Triangle*, paper presented at the Conference of the National Association for Clean Air, Dikholo, South Africa

von Schinrding, Y E R, Yach, D and Klein, M (1991a) 'Acute respiratory infections as an important cause of childhood deaths in South Africa' in *South African Medical Journal*, vol 80, no 2, pp79–82

von Schirnding, Y E R, Yach, D, Blignaut, R and Mathews, C (1991b) 'Environmental determinants of acute respiratory symptoms and diarrhoea in young coloured children living in urban and peri-urban areas of South Africa' in *South African Medical Journal*, vol 79, no 8, pp457–461

von Schirnding, Y, Bradshaw, D, Fuggle, R and Stokol, M (1991c) 'Blood lead levels in South African inner-city children' in *Environmental Health Perspectives*, vol 94, pp125–130

von Schirnding, Y E R and Mokoetle, K (1993) 'Soweto child health mortality study: preliminary results at 6 months' in *Urbanisation and Health Newsletter*, vol 17, pp58–61

von Schirnding, Y E and Fuggle, R F (1996) 'A study of the distribution of urban environmental lead levels in Cape Town, South Africa' in *Science of the Total Environment*, vol 20, no 188(1), pp1–8

Yach, D, Cameron, N, Padayachee, N, Wagstaff, L, Richter, L and Fonn, S (1991) 'Birth to ten: child health in South Africa in the 1990s: rationale and methods of a birth cohort study' in *Paediatric and Perinatal Epidemiology*, vol 5, no 2, pp211–233

Index

For Product Safety Concerns and Information please contact our EU
representative GPSR@taylorandfrancis.com Taylor & Francis Verlag GmbH,
Kaufingerstraße 24, 80331 München, Germany

Printed and bound by CPI Group (UK) Ltd, Croydon, CR0 4YY

01/05/2025

01858505-0001